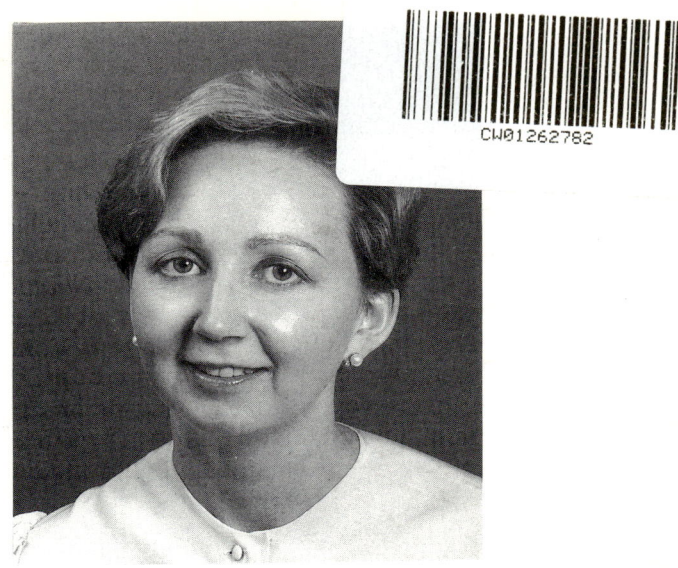

Anne Szarewski DRCOG, trained initially at the Middlesex Hospital Medical School, London and then in Obstetrics and Gynaecology at the Royal Northern and Whittington Hospitals. She is currently a Research Fellow in Gynaecological Oncology involved in a study of cervical precancer. She is an Instructing Doctor in Family Planning at the Margaret Pyke Centre, London, and also at the Marie Stopes Clinic in London.

OPTIMA

HORMONAL CONTRACEPTION
A WOMAN'S GUIDE

Dr Anne Szarewski

Illustrated by Jennie Smith

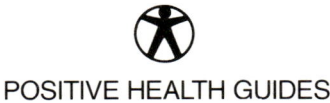
POSITIVE HEALTH GUIDES

An OPTIMA book

© Dr Anne Szarewski 1991

First published in 1991 by
Macdonald Optima, a division of
Macdonald & Co. (Publishers) Ltd

A member of Maxwell Macmillan Pergamon Publishing Corporation

All rights reserved

No part of this publication may be reproduced,
stored in a retrieval system, or transmitted,
in any form or by any means without the prior
permission in writing of the publisher, nor be
otherwise circulated in any form of binding or
cover other than that in which it is published
and without a similar condition including this
condition being imposed on the subsequent
purchaser.

British Library Cataloguing in Publication Data

Szarewski, Anne
    Hormonal contraception.
    1. Oral contraceptives
    I. Title
    613.9432

    ISBN 0-356-19556-2

Macdonald & Co. (Publishers) Ltd
Orbit House
1 New Fetter Lane
London EC4A 1AR

Typeset in Times by Leaper & Gard Ltd, Bristol

Printed and bound in Great Britain by
BPCC Hazell Books
Aylesbury, Bucks, England
Member of BPCC Ltd.

CONTENTS

	Acknowledgements	vi
	Introduction	vii
1	Female hormones, the reproductive process and the development of hormonal contraception	1
2	The Combined Pill — risks and benefits	17
3	Which pill should I take? Dealing with side effects	35
4	Taking the Pill — the practicalities	60
5	The Progestogen-Only Pill	75
6	Injectable progestogens	89
7	Hormonal contraception at special times	100
8	Hormonal contraception in the future	112
9	Hormonal contraception for men	123
10	The pros and cons of hormonal contraception	133
	Further reading	136
	Useful addresses	138

ACKNOWLEDGEMENTS

My main debt of gratitude must go to Mr John Guillebaud, Medical Director of the Margaret Pyke Centre in London. It was his teaching which first inspired me to enter the field of family planning, and his book *The Pill* which confirmed my tentatively held view that detailed medical information could be presented in a form that most people would understand. We do not necessarily always hold the same views, and opinions I give in this book should not automatically be assumed to also be his, nor the official policy of the Margaret Pyke Centre. However, he has been a constant source of guidance, information and support. I would also like to thank him for reading the manuscript and making useful comments.

I would like to thank Dr Jack Cuzick of the Imperial Cancer Research Fund for reading and commenting on the sections dealing with breast and cervical cancer. I would also like to thank my editor, Ms Harriet Griffey, and the other staff at Optima who have always been encouraging and supportive. Lastly, I would like to thank my family, friends and colleagues who have had to put up with my distracted air, my stubborn hibernation at weekends and my frequent announcements of how the book was or was not progressing!

INTRODUCTION

We still do not have a perfect method of contraception. Such a method would provide complete protection against pregnancy, be entirely free from health risks and side effects, not involve any action either during or immediately prior to intercourse, be completely reversible, not rely on the user's memory, and not involve the medical profession. It seems unlikely that this goal will be reached for a very long time to come.

Meanwhile, we have a variety of different, less-than-perfect methods. They all have advantages and drawbacks. In general, it can be said that the more effective a method is, the more likely it is to have health risks or side effects. Similarly, if a method is relatively free of health risks, it is likely to be less effective at preventing pregnancy.

In the end, each couple has to balance the risks and the benefits, bearing their own medical histories and lifestyle in mind. These may change over time, and therefore they may wish to use several different methods at different times.

This book is about hormonal methods of contraception. In general, these are the more effective methods at preventing pregnancy, but by the same token, they may have health risks and side effects. Many of these can be avoided or at least reduced if the right method is chosen for a particular woman, and many of the side effects can be minimised if you know how to deal with them, and what to expect.

Many women feel that they are not able to make a rational decision about hormonal methods because they do not have enough information. The benefits and risks of the sheath, for example, are relatively straightforward, and most people are aware of them. Hormonal contraception is much more complicated and therefore requires more thought. In addition, hormonal methods are often the subject of press reports, which may be sensationalised and make it more difficult to have an unbiased view.

In this book I hope to present the facts, and dispel some of the myths which have accumulated over the years. If I succeed, you should find it easier to reach a decision about what is best for you. I also hope it will help women who are already using a hormonal method of contraception and are having problems. Ignorance breeds fear, and there are many quite simple problems which nevertheless cause a great deal of unnecessary anxiety.

Contraception should involve both partners, not just the woman. In the future, hormonal contraception may be available for men, bringing a new meaning to the equality of the sexes. Chapter 9 looks at the options which look most promising.

I have tried to make the chapters as self-contained as possible, so that you can 'dip into' the book as well as read it straight through. However, most readers will find it helpful to read Chapter 1, since this is where I discuss many basic concepts which it is impossible to keep repeating in full later on.

1

FEMALE HORMONES, THE REPRODUCTIVE PROCESS AND THE DEVELOPMENT OF HORMONAL CONTRACEPTION

In order to understand how hormonal methods of contraception work, we must first look at the way a woman's natural hormones interact. We need to start off in the brain, and in particular, in an area called the hypothalamus. The hypothalamus controls the release of a hormone called Gonadotrophin Releasing Hormone, or GnRH for short ('Gonad' means 'sex organ' and 'trophic' derives from the Greek for 'to nourish or stimulate', so the name means 'hormone which causes the release of something which stimulates the sex organs' – 'GnRH' is much quicker, you will agree). GnRH passes down to the pituitary gland, where it causes the release of two more hormones, Follicle Stimulating Hormone (FSH) and Luteinising Hormone (LH). These enter the bloodstream and make their way to the ovaries.

When a female baby is born, her ovaries already contain millions of little fluid-filled 'bubbles' or follicles, each of which is potentially able to develop into an ovum, or egg. No more are ever formed: on the contrary, they keep disappearing all the time, so that by puberty, only about 200,000 are left. I say 'only', but of course, this is still far more than any woman could ever need.

FSH, as its name suggests, acts to stimulate a group of these 'bubbles' or follicles to grow. One follicle will grow more quickly than the others, and it is this one which is destined to

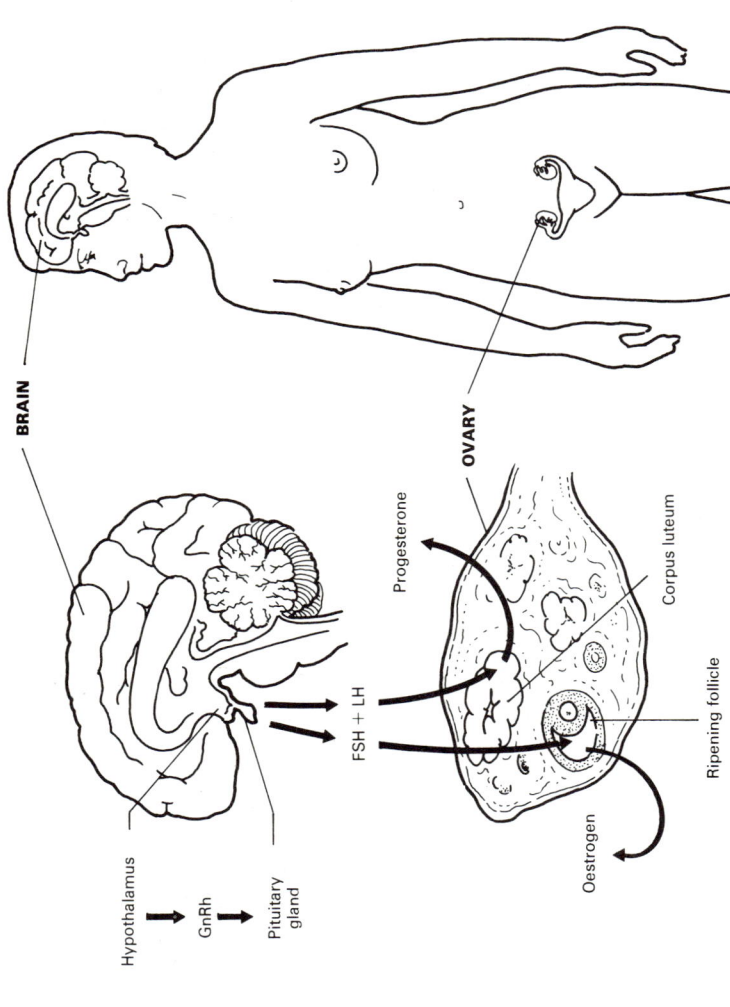

Figure 1.1 Hormones released from the brain stimulate the release of hormones from the ovary which in turn feed back to the brain.

actually become an ovum or egg. As the follicles grow, they release oestrogen, which again enters the bloodstream and is carried all around the body. It is oestrogen which makes women look like women, causing the breasts to grow, and the body to take on a more rounded shape than is seen in men.

Oestrogen has many effects all around the body, but also goes back to the brain. When it reaches the pituitary gland two things happen. First of all, high levels of oestrogen halt the production of FSH, thereby stopping the situation from going out of control. This is called 'negative feedback' and acts a little like the thermostat which controls a central heating system: when the temperature in the house reaches a certain level, the thermostat switches the heating off for a while, so that the house does not become too hot. When the temperature drops, the thermostat switches the heating on again, and so on. Many hormones are controlled in this way in the body, such that high levels of a hormone cause a 'switching off' of the mechanism which leads to its production or release (see Figure 1.1).

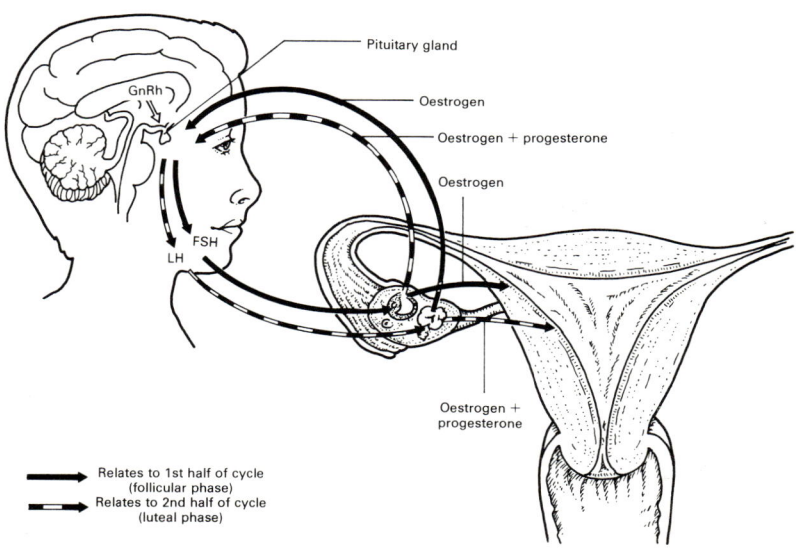

Figure 1.2 Effect of ovarian hormones on the pituitary gland.

3

The oestrogen which reaches the pituitary gland has another more unusual effect: when it reaches a certain level, it actually causes a sudden *rise* in the release of LH. This is called 'positive feedback', in that the situation is being encouraged to go 'out of control'. This LH 'surge', as it is called, rushes back down to the ovaries and causes the largest 'bubble' or follicle to burst, releasing an ovum (egg).

Once an egg has been released, the remaining follicles resign themselves to their disappointment and get down to the serious business of helping the egg survive in the hope of meeting a sperm. The follicles, under the influence of LH, form a small yellow area in the ovary, called the 'corpus luteum', which simply means 'yellow body' in Latin (but doesn't it sound so much more important in a foreign language?). In fact, the name Luteinising Hormone really just means 'the hormone which causes the yellowness to happen'.

The corpus luteum then starts to produce large quantities of another hormone, progesterone, in addition to oestrogen. Like oestrogen, progesterone has effects throughout the body, but its main function is to make the uterus (womb) into a comfortable bed for the hopefully by now fertilised egg. ('Progesterone' derives from 'pro-gestation', which means 'towards pregnancy'). It does this in two ways. Firstly, it makes the lining of the womb nice and thick (rather like a soft mattress). Secondly, it increases the number of glands in the lining: these produce a fluid which both makes the lining more comfortable and provides the potential embryo with nourishment.

If the egg is indeed fertilised, the embryo settles itself (or implants) into this warm nest in the womb, and then prepares to fight for its life: it has to prevent its nest being ripped off and washed away with the next period. Its main weapon is a hormone which it produces, called Human Chorionic Gonadotrophin (HCG). This acts like a runner, telling the corpus luteum to keep sending the supplies of oestrogen and particularly progesterone, which keep the lining thick and prevent it from coming off. In addition, HCG lets the pituitary know that these high levels of oestrogen and progesterone are meant to support the embryo, not to cause another surge of LH (otherwise another egg could be released and a woman could become pregnant while already pregnant).

Even with such elaborate preparations and defences, this battle is very often lost. Many very early pregnancies do not manage to survive and are simply knocked off the wall of the womb and washed away as the lining disappears in the next period. In this situation, and also if the egg is not fertilised, the corpus luteum just packs up and disappears. This leads to a sudden drop in both oestrogen and progesterone, causing the glands in the womb to shrivel up and the lining to come off the walls, resulting in a period. Meanwhile, the other effect of the drop in oestrogen and progesterone levels is that the thermostat switches on the production of FSH again, which stimulates another group of follicles, and the whole process is repeated. This is called the menstrual cycle.

In actual fact, there are several other hormones involved. For example, in addition to oestrogen, the follicles also produce a hormone called inhibin, which specifically blocks the action of FSH (another negative feedback mechanism). We shall be mentioning inhibin later in this book, particularly in connection with research into finding a male pill. The hormone prolactin, whose main function is the production of milk during breast-feeding, also gets involved, as do just about all the hormones which travel around in the bloodstream. In fact, the process is so complex that very few doctors really understand it, and there are certainly many unanswered questions which are the subject of a great deal of research. However, it is not necessary to be a top scientist to understand basically what goes on and to grasp the principle of the menstrual cycle.

The so-called 'normal' menstrual cycle lasts 28 days, from the first day of a period to the first day of the next one. However, in women who are not taking hormones, this 'normal' cycle is a myth. Many women have longer or shorter cycles, which vary in length from month to month, and are completely normal. The length of the cycle can be influenced by many things. Starting at the top again, it is obvious that the brain is closely involved in the whole process. This is why travelling, stress or a sudden shock can disrupt a woman's periods, or even stop them altogether for a time – and yet be entirely 'natural'.

There is only one fixed time interval in the cycle, which is that the next period will come 14 days after the egg has been released, if pregnancy does not occur and continue. This is the length of time it takes for the corpus luteum to disappear and for the lining to start to come away. It is the reason why the 'rhythm' method of family planning is so prone to failure: the date of ovulation is always only known in retrospect, never in advance. The only women who do in fact know when they are ovulating are those who experience pain as the follicle bursts, releasing the egg. This is because a little blood may be spilt at the same time, which irritates the surrounding tissues and causes pain. This pain is given the technical name of 'mittelschmerz' ('pain in the middle' obviously sounds more scientific in

German). Of course, the pain only occurs exactly at mid-cycle if the woman does have 28-day cycles, otherwise it will simply occur 14 days prior to the next period.

You may ask, 'Why is it possible to become pregnant in the first half of the cycle, if everything important actually happens in the second half?' The answer is that sperm thought of that before you did. Unfortunately (or fortunately, depending on how you look at it) sperm can survive in the uterus (womb) and fallopian tubes for four or five days, occasionally even a week. This means that even if you have sex several days before you ovulate, the sperm can be sitting waiting, ready to pounce.

Incidentally, you may not have realised that the very sensitive pregnancy tests which have become available in the last few years are based on the detection of the hormone HCG, produced by the embryo itself. Levels of HCG get higher and higher as time passes, and these tests are often capable of detecting a pregnancy by the time of the missed period, sometimes even before. This is a mixed blessing, however. As we have seen, many early pregnancies do not manage to survive, and are washed away as a normal or slightly late period. A lot of anxiety (or false hope) can be caused by such early detection of pregnancy, which then comes to nothing.

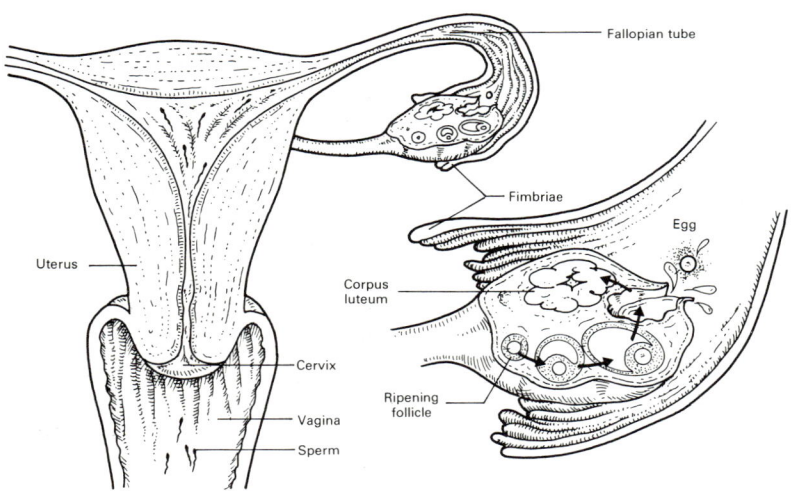

Figure 1.3 The orum (egg) is released from the ovary and guided down the fallopian tube. The sperm travel up the vagina and into the uterus and fallopian tubes where conception can occur.

Let's just run through the reproductive process quickly again, thinking more about the anatomy this time. When an ovum (egg) is released from the ovary, it is literally sucked into the waiting, open end of the fallopian tube. The finger-like extensions at the end of the tube are called fimbriae. Inside the tube there are many little hairs called cilia, which help to move the egg along the tube into the uterus (womb) itself.

Meanwhile, during sex, millions of sperm are deposited in the vagina when the man ejaculates (but some will also enter before this, which is why withdrawal is not a very effective method of contraception). The vagina is an acidic environment, which sperm do not like, so they have to try and get into the uterus, via the cervix, as quickly as possible. If they stay too long in the vagina they will die.

The woman makes life easier for the sperm, because when she is sexually excited, especially around mid-cycle, glands in the vagina and cervical canal produce a particularly sperm-friendly mucus, which is long and stretchy, and can actually act a little like a ladder into the uterus. Also, it is thought that during orgasm, the sperm are actively sucked into the uterus. This is the basis for the popular myth that if a woman does not have an orgasm, she will not become pregnant. However, with so many millions of sperm, one is still likely to get through even without extra help.

Sperm which enter the vagina are still not fully active and do not have the capacity to fertilise an egg. While they are travelling through the mucus, they become fully activated, and this process is called 'capacitation' (i.e. they now have the capacity to fertilise). Some new approaches to 'male' contraception are looking into ways of blocking this capacitation – I say 'male contraception' with some irony as, of course, such methods would have to be used by women....

Once sperm are actually inside the uterus they can relax. This is a very pleasant environment for them, and it is here that they can happily live for several days. Some of them will swim their way into the fallopian tubes, and may meet an egg there. Fertilisation can, and indeed often does occur in a fallopian tube, but the embryo normally moves into the main part of the uterus before implanting itself into the specially prepared, thick lining. If for some reason it implants itself while still in the tube, it becomes an ectopic pregnancy (in Greek, 'ecto' means 'outside' and 'topos' means 'place', i.e. a pregnancy outside the right place). An embryo may settle in the tube if, for example, the little hairs, or cilia, in the tube are damaged and do not move it into the uterus fast enough. This is most likely to be caused by an infection of the tubes (salpingitis, or pelvic inflammatory disease), and is the reason why intrauterine contraceptive devices (IUDs), which make tubal infection more likely, are also associated with a greater chance of having an ectopic pregnancy.

An ectopic pregnancy is dangerous because, as you know, pregnancies get bigger and bigger, and need space to expand. The uterus is an ideal place, as it is specifically designed to grow when a woman is pregnant. The tubes are not, and will therefore burst when the pregnancy becomes too big. When that happens, the woman's life is in danger due to internal bleeding and the risk of subsequent infection.

Anyway, let us assume that fertilisation has taken place and the embryo is safely inside the uterus. As we saw earlier, it now implants itself in the lining of the uterus, and hopes to survive.

Contraceptive methods have to block this process somewhere along the line, and most of them act in several different ways, to increase the chances of success. For example, methods such as the diaphragm and sheath act as physical barriers, on the basis that if you can stop sperm from getting into the cervix, they will soon die in the vagina. However, they are usually recommended for use with spermicides, designed to actively kill or immobilise sperm, in case the physical barrier is not enough. The IUD nowadays usually contains copper, which seems to act as a sort of poison to try and prevent fertilisation in the first place, but if that fails, to kill the fertilised embryo before it implants, and lastly, to actually disrupt the implantation process so that it is unsuccessful.

Hormonal methods in general interfere with earlier stages of the process, by preventing or disrupting ovulation. However, they often also have 'back-up' mechanisms further down the line, which they rely on to a lesser or greater extent.

The Combined Pill works by preventing ovulation from happening, by literally fooling the brain into thinking that the woman is pregnant. It does this by capitalising on the negative feedback process which is already set up naturally. You may remember that in pregnancy, the high levels of oestrogen and progesterone tell the pituitary gland to stop producing FSH and LH. This ensures that the woman does not ovulate a second time when she is already pregnant.

The levels of the two hormones in the pill are high enough to make the brain think that the woman must be pregnant, and therefore it stops producing FSH and LH, and ovulation does not occur. It is remarkably simple. The pill also thickens cervical mucus, making it less easy for sperm to get through, but this has little importance once ovulation has been blocked – there is no egg waiting even if they do get through.

HOW HORMONAL CONTRACEPTION WAS DEVELOPED

Hormonal contraception is not a new idea, although the earliest experimenters did not realise that was what they were trying to achieve. Many ancient civilisations have advocated swallowing things as contraceptives, rather than using barriers. For example, in China they suggested that women should swallow live tadpoles! In India, various potions were proposed, including large quantities of three-year-old molasses to be eaten every day for a fortnight. Any woman who managed to do this was supposed to remain childless for the rest of her life. Another way of becoming permanently childless was to drink a potion made up of the Kallambha plant mixed with the feet of jungle flies. In Europe in the thirteenth century, St Albert suggested that live bees should be eaten – one has to wonder whether this was actually meant as a punishment for attempting to use contraception.

Almost every culture has used plant-derived mixtures in order to try and prevent pregnancy, and although the vast majority were probably useless, if not dangerous, it is likely that some really worked. Scientists have for many years been studying these herbal medicines, and some have been shown to contain hormones, or substances which would have been likely to induce a miscarriage.

It is therefore not entirely surprising to find that we owe modern hormonal contraception to the Mexican yam. The roots of these yams contain a substance called diosgenin, from which it was found to be possible to produce progesterone. This was a major breakthrough, because until then all hormones had had to be obtained from animals. The time and expense this involved had seriously impeded the progress of research in this area – both oestrogen and progesterone had been isolated by the early 1930s, but they were of little practical use while it required literally tens of thousands of animals to produce enough hormone for one human dose. In 1941, the Mexican yam changed all that, and made the production of an oral contraceptive pill a realistic proposition for the first time. Mexico proved an even better source of raw materials when it was later discovered that the root of a different plant contained up to ten times as much diosgenin as the yam.

At first, the hormone had to be given by injection – so in fact, progesterone by injection was the very first method of hormonal contraception to be developed. It was quickly realised that a pill would be much more widely acceptable, and the large quantities of hormone now available meant that research progressed by leaps and bounds. By 1953 the first contraceptive pills were ready, largely financed and encouraged by two American women, Margaret Sanger and Katherine McCormick. These enthusiastic campaigners for women's rights were responsible, more than anyone else, for making the pill available to women. You must remember that at the time contraception was a taboo subject, and pharmaceutical companies were not very keen to be seen promoting it. There was always the possibility that their other products would be boycotted in a campaign against them, thus putting them rapidly out of business.

At first, the new pills were put on trial as a treatment for period problems – something for which the pill is still used today. They contained high doses of what was thought to be pure progestogen, and worked very well. Women took them for three weeks and then had a week's break: bleeding patterns were very acceptable and there were few complaints of side effects.

As the production process of the pills was improved, the contents were purified still further. Suddenly, the newer pills were found to be less effective and to cause irregular bleeding. The companies found that they had to reintroduce a substance which they had thought was an unnecessary contaminant: oestrogen. Once they realised this, they started putting in specific quantities of oestrogen, thus creating the Combined Pill.

This pill, however, bore little resemblance to the one we know today. It contained 150 micrograms of oestrogen and 10 milligrams of progestogen. Modern pills usually contain around 30 micrograms of oestrogen and one milligram of that type of progestogen. So you can see that the dose of oestrogen is now only a fifth, while the dose of progestogen is a tenth of what was being used in the 1960s.

Nowadays, women tend to voice complaints about the pill if they put on a couple of pounds in weight, or have a few headaches: it is a reflection of the need of women in the 1960s that they welcomed this high-dose preparation so enthusiastically. Prior to the pill, the only methods available were caps and sheaths (and then only to married women). Early pill users must have put on large amounts of weight, probably needed bras a couple of sizes larger than before, and had a myriad of other side effects. And yet they stayed on it, and it grew in popularity, such was the need for an effective method of contraception.

The 'honeymoon' lasted till 1968, when the first reports were published which showed that women who took the pill were more likely to have a blood clot in a vein (venous thrombosis). In itself, this is unpleasant, but the real danger lies in the fact that such a clot can become dislodged and travel in the circulation to the lungs. If it sticks there and disrupts the blood flow in the lungs, a pulmonary embolism is said to have occurred. This can be life-threatening.

Not surprisingly, there was an enormous pill scare. For the first time, women and their doctors realised that taking the pill was not as simple and safe as it had seemed. There was a price to be paid for everything.

The pharmaceutical companies rushed off and produced pills containing less oestrogen. At the time, it was thought that oestrogen was the sole culprit in terms of health risks, and so they reduced the dose to 50 micrograms, while retaining very high doses of progestogen. Everything went well again for several years, until it was shown that the dose of progestogen was just as important. A study was published which showed that if women took pills containing the same dose of oestrogen, but different doses of progestogen, their risks of clots and other circulatory diseases depended on the dose of progestogen. Once again there was a pill scare, and once again the pharmaceutical companies went off and produced pills with lower doses, this time of progestogen.

During the last ten years, there have been so many pill scares that doctors in family planning have begun to regard them as an occupational hazard. Some have been justified, some not. However, as a result of the increasing concern over the safety of the pill, an enormous amount of research has gone into producing lower and lower-dose pills, and into refining the hormones still further in an effort to reduce side effects and health risks. In order to better understand these developments, we must now look at the functions of oestrogen and progesterone in the body, and then see how they relate to the effects of the hormones used in the pill.

THE FUNCTIONS OF OESTROGEN AND PROGESTERONE

These two hormones are central to female development. They have many complicated actions throughout the body, not all of which are understood. The explanations given here will be, of necessity, simplified, but should be enough to allow you to understand later many of the actions and side effects of hormonal contraceptives.

Oestrogen

Oestrogen (which is really a family of hormones) has the prime function of causing the development of the female sex organs, and the so-called 'secondary' sexual characteristics of the female. These are, for example, the breasts, the distribution of body hair in women, and, regrettably for many of us, the distribution of fat around the body.

As we have already seen, oestrogen is responsible for many stages in the menstrual cycle. It promotes the growth of the endometrium (lining of the womb) in the first half of the cycle, and makes the fimbriae (end) of the fallopian tube move towards the ovarian follicle, to help guide the ovum (egg) into the tube. It helps make muscles contract, thereby aiding, among other things, the movement of the ovum down the tube into the uterus (womb).

It causes an increase in libido (sex drive) at mid-cycle, and, also at mid-cycle, makes the cervical mucus become particularly sperm-friendly. The mucus becomes thinner and therefore easier for the sperm to move through in order to reach the cervix.

Oestrogen is also important in making the skin supple and elastic. This applies throughout the body, but also in the vagina, making it easier for it to expand in pregnancy, and also giving it the elasticity necessary for intercourse.

Oestrogen has a tendency to cause water retention by increasing the retention of salt. It also stimulates the production of a number of hormones by the liver. For our purposes, the important ones are:

- Sex Hormone Binding Globulin (increased)
- High-density lipoproteins (increased)
- Various factors which are involved in blood clotting

High-density lipoproteins (also known as HDL cholesterol), which are blood fats, are protective against atherosclerosis (the so-called 'hardening of the arteries'). This means that oestrogen acts to protect women from the risks of cardiovascular disease. This protective effect is further enhanced by the fact that oestrogen tends to cause a decrease in low-density lipoproteins (also called LDL cholesterol). LDL cholesterol acts in opposition to HDL cholesterol and therefore tends to increase the risk of cardiovascular disease. This can be neatly summed up by the phrase 'HDL good, LDL bad'. Since oestrogen both increases HDL and decreases LDL, it is clearly, from this point of view, very good.

I shall discuss Sex Hormone Binding Globulin in the next section, on the actions of progestogens.

The other very important function of oestrogen is that it helps maintain the structure of bones. After the menopause, when production of oestrogen by the ovaries stops, women tend to develop osteoporosis. This is a condition in which, because of the lack of oestrogen, bone material is actually lost from the body. Obviously, this makes the bones thinner and more liable to break. In addition, because of bone loss in the spine, women actually become shorter in old age. Oestrogen deficiency is a major cause of both physical and psychological ill-health in women after the menopause. Nowadays, however, the importance of oestrogen has been recognised, and hormone replacement therapy has been developed to try, as its name suggests, to replace the oestrogen which the body is losing, and to prevent the changes which would otherwise occur in both bones and skin.

Progesterone

Progesterone is the hormone which is mainly responsible for preparing the body for pregnancy. As we have seen, it, like oestrogen, plays an important part in the menstrual cycle, particularly in the second half, where its main function is to keep the lining of the womb nice and thick to help a pregnancy survive.

Progesterone, in conjunction with another hormone, prolactin, stimulates the breasts in preparation for the production of milk.

Progesterone, in contrast to oestrogen, makes cervical mucus thick and more difficult for sperm to penetrate.

Once again, in contrast to oestrogen, progesterone tends to lead to a loss of salt from the body, and therefore to a loss of water.

Natural progesterone is destroyed in the stomach, and therefore cannot be given by mouth. The eagle-eyed among you will probably have noticed that, half-way through the account of the development of the pill, I subtly stopped talking about progesterone and started talking about progestogen instead.

Progestogens

Progestogens are synthetic compounds and, although they have many things in common with progesterone, there are also many differences. These differences mostly stem from the compounds from which progestogens are derived.

Most progestogens are derived from testosterone, which is the male sex hormone. This is not as ridiculous as it sounds. The difference between male and female hormones is not that great, and you will later see that in fact, 'female' hormones are being used in the development of the 'male pill'. In addition, all women do, in fact, have a small amount of testosterone normally circulating in their bodies.

The only problem with the synthesis of progestogens from testosterone is that it proved remarkably difficult to remove absolutely all the 'male' characteristics. This means that these synthetic progestogens did not have exactly the same effects in the body as progesterone: they have also had so-called 'androgenic' effects. Broadly speaking, the term 'androgenic' is used to describe male characteristics as applied to women. Thus we can explain why progestogens are normally associated with side effects such as excess hair and acne. In addition, they can cause weight gain because they can increase the appetite (remember oestrogen can cause weight gain, but by increasing water retention). In some women, these progestogens can reduce libido.

The other very important effect of progestogens is that they lower HDL cholesterol and raise LDL cholesterol. This is bad, as it promotes the development of cardiovascular disease.

Earlier I mentioned that oestrogens increase the production of Sex Hormone Binding Globulin (SHBG) by the liver. SHBG tends to 'mop up' circulating testosterone and progestogens, thus diminishing so-called 'androgenic' side effects (acne, excess hair, etc.). However, progestogens themselves counteract the rise in SHBG caused by oestrogen, thus tending to increase these types of side effects. I shall be mentioning SHBG again later, when I discuss the link between the Combined Pill and breast cancer (see Chapter 2).

You may have noticed that I seem to be torn between the present and past tense in this discussion of progestogens. And there is a very good reason. In the last few years, a new 'generation' of progestogens have been produced, which behave quite differently from the ones we have had so far. In the simplest terms, the scientists finally managed to get rid of the irritating 'male' aspects of progestogens, thereby overturning everything which I have said about progestogens so far.

These new progestogens are described as 'highly specific', which means that they do not have the unwanted 'androgenic' side effects of the older ones. Before we go any further, you need to understand an important concept:

Oestrogens and progestogens in the pill interact with each other, and therefore the actual effects seen will depend on the doses of both hormones as well as the exact type of progestogen. In this context, it is pointless to view them on their own.

What this means in practice is that certain combinations will tend to produce an overall 'oestrogenic bias' or 'dominance' while others will produce an overall 'progestogenic bias' or 'dominance'. This will, to a great extent, govern the type of side effects a woman experiences on a particular brand, and may also affect potential health risks.

In pill brands containing the older progestogens, oestrogen and progestogen 'fight' each other, since they tend to have opposing effects. The characteristics of that brand will then depend on which of the two is 'stronger'. This effect is greatly reduced in pill brands which contain the new progestogens, since they are basically 'wimps' with very few, if any, 'androgenic' effects.

Modern pills (i.e. with less than 40 micrograms of oestrogen) which contain the older progestogens tend to have the effect of slightly lowering a woman's HDL cholesterol. Although this is not desirable, the effect is very small. They usually also tend to slightly lower Sex Hormone Binding Globulin (SHBG), which again is not desirable, as it potentially increases the 'androgenic' side effects.

The newest pills, containing the latest progestogens (which are desogestrel, gestodene and soon norgestimate) do not have these effects. In fact, they behave almost as though the progestogen was not there at all. So women using these pills have normal, even slightly raised levels of HDL cholesterol and SHBG.

It has to be said, however, that in the extremely low pill doses which we have reached in the late 1980s and 1990s, these effects are much less significant, and there are sceptics who question whether these new 'wonder' progestogens will make a great deal of difference. Ever since the dose of hormones was reduced to current levels, the number of serious health risks due to the pill has been extremely small, and it may well be that further improvements will not have much significance. However, what is emerging is that these newer formulations have fewer of the 'niggling', so-called 'minor' side effects, which are not at all 'minor' to the women who experience them. It is in this area that I think the newest pills have their greatest advantage. The differences between individual formulations are discussed in detail in Chapter 3. Meanwhile, let us look at the risks and benefits of being on the pill.

2

THE COMBINED PILL – RISKS AND BENEFITS

Over 60 million women currently take the pill, and 150 million are estimated to have used it since it was introduced. No other medication has been taken regularly by so many women, nor has any medication been studied so closely. Taking the pill is associated with both risks and benefits, which in each individual case need to be balanced against each other. Every woman has a different family history, medical history, lifestyle and set of particular worries. These all need to be taken into account when making a decision about any form of contraception, not just the pill.

We all hear so much about the risks of the pill, one sometimes wonders how it is that the entire female population has not been wiped out since it was introduced. I would like to start by introducing you to a rarely mentioned concept: the pill can be good for you, too.

HEALTH BENEFITS OF THE PILL

Prevention of pregnancy

This may not strike you immediately as a health benefit, but it is a very important one. The pill has a failure rate of only about 0.5 to 1 per 100 women years, which means that if 200 women take it for a year, only one or at most two will become pregnant accidentally.

Few people think of pregnancy as a dangerous time, but in fact, in many countries in the developing world it is the most important cause of death in women. Even in this country, being pregnant is nearly 10 times more dangerous to your health than being on the pill, if you are young and do not smoke. Even if you do smoke, if you are under 35 your risk from the pill is only the same as if you were pregnant.

Prevention of ectopic pregnancy

Because the pill stops you ovulating and is so effective, it also gives virtually complete protection from ectopic pregnancy. An ectopic pregnancy is a pregnancy in the fallopian tube (see Chapter 1), and can be a life-threatening condition. Even if you survive, it has been estimated that about two-thirds of women are then infertile.

Protection against pelvic inflammatory disease (PID)

Women using the pill have only half the risk of developing PID (also called salpingitis) compared with non-users. This is likely to be due to its effect on cervical mucus: if sperm cannot get through, 'germs' are less likely to as well. PID is a major cause of infertility, so once again paradoxically, taking the pill can actually protect your fertility.

Fewer problems with periods

The pill is very effective in relieving dysmenorrhoea (period pain). Indeed, it has been shown to help 90 per cent of women who have painful periods.

The pill also reduces the heaviness of blood flow during periods, which apart from the obvious practical advantages helps to prevent women becoming anaemic. It has been shown that women on the pill lose only about half as much iron from their blood because of the reduction in menstrual flow.

Relief from premenstrual syndrome (PMS)

Women who take monophasic pills (which have the same dose all month) usually find that their PMS symptoms are much improved by the pill. This is not so often the case if triphasic pills are used (see Chapter 3).

Prevention of ovarian cysts

The pill gives about a 90 per cent protection against the development of non-cancerous ovarian cysts. Although these are not usually dangerous they can rupture and lead to pain and hospitalisation. The pill has this protective effect by making the ovaries inactive, and therefore less likely to produce cysts. Indeed, the pill is sometimes used as a treatment for a condition known as 'polycystic ovary syndrome' in which the ovaries form a large number of small cysts; by making the ovaries inactive, the pill stops the formation of these cysts, and leads to an improvement.

Prevention of benign breast disease

The pill gives a 50 to 75 per cent reduction in benign breast disease (also called mastitis). It means you are less likely to develop benign (non-cancerous) breast lumps, or to develop lumpy, tender areas. This is an important effect, because it very significantly reduces the number of women who have to have breast biopsies taken, a procedure which is both unpleasant and traumatic for the woman concerned.

Reduced likelihood of developing fibroids

Fibroids are swellings of the muscle which makes up the womb. They are more common in women of African or West Indian origin, though the reason for this is not known. Although they do not become cancerous, they can grow to the size of a football. If they become large, they start to cause problems because of their sheer size. They can make you feel fat, because they can actually cause a visible swelling. They can press on the bladder resulting in a need to pass urine more frequently. They can cause constipation by pressing on the bowel. They are also associated with an increased chance of having a miscarriage.

The pill actually makes women about 30 per cent less likely to develop fibroids. In addition, if you are beginning to develop one, then the pill can slow down its growth. In such cases a 'progestogen-dominant' pill (see Chapter 3) should be used.

Relieving the symptoms of endometriosis

Endometriosis is an unpleasant gynaecological condition which results in very painful, heavy periods, as well as pain before and after the period. There are various treatments for endometriosis which are more effective at curing it than the pill, but the pill can certainly help by removing the symptoms associated with periods. Also, not all women can tolerate the side effects of the more effective treatments. In such cases, the pill should be taken without any breaks, to avoid bleeding, and a 'progestogen-dominant' brand (see Chapter 3) should be used.

Reduced risk of duodenal ulcers

Several studies have suggested that women who use the pill are less likely to suffer from duodenal ulcers. This has not been studied in detail, so we cannot yet be sure that this is true.

Reduction in rheumatoid arthritis

A large study has suggested that pill users are protected against rheumatoid arthritis by a factor of 50 per cent. Once again, this needs to be confirmed by other studies before we can be sure it is true.

Improvements in skin and hair

The pill can greatly improve acne, and indeed is often used by dermatologists as a treatment for acne. It can also help stop the growth of excess hair on the body (hirsutism) and improve greasy hair. In all these cases, an 'oestrogen-dominant' pill should be used (see Chapter 3), preferably containing one of the new progestogens, e.g. Marvelon.

Protection against ovarian cancer

It has been established that the pill gives a 40 per cent reduction in the chance of developing ovarian cancer. The even better news is that you only have to take the pill for a year to be protected, and the protection lasts for many years – as it would have to, since ovarian cancer is most common in women over 50. It has been shown that the protective effect is true for both the older high-dose pills and the lower-dose ones used in recent years. This is a very important health benefit of the pill, since ovarian cancer is a major cause of death in older women: about twice as many die of ovarian cancer as of cervical cancer.

Protection against endometrial cancer

As with ovarian cancer, it is well established that the pill gives a 50 per cent reduction in the risk of developing cancer of the endometrium (the body of the womb, as opposed to the cervix, or neck of the womb). Once again, you only have to take the pill for a year to be protected, and the effect lasts for many years. Endometrial cancer is also most common in women over the age of 50. Again, as for ovarian cancer, the protective effect holds for both high- and low-dose pills.

The protective effects of the pill against both ovarian and endometrial cancer are very strong, and proven beyond doubt. It is interesting that both these cancers have the same risk factors (i.e. things which make a woman more likely to develop them). It is known that a woman is more likely to develop both these cancers if she starts to have periods young (under 12), stops having them late, i.e. has a late menopause, does not have children, and never takes the pill. The factor which all those things have in common is periods. It seems that the more periods a woman has in her lifetime (and therefore the more often she ovulates), the more likely she is to develop ovarian and endometrial cancer. What is even more interesting is that the risk factors for breast cancer are exactly the same. It is therefore puzzling that not only does the pill not appear to give any protection against breast cancer, but has even, in some studies, appeared to increase the risk. We will be looking into this in more detail in the next section.

THE POSSIBLE HEALTH RISKS OF THE PILL

Cardiovascular disease (heart and blood vessels)

The effect of the pill on blood clotting was the first reported serious health risk, in the 1960s. At first, scientists believed that the risk was all due to the oestrogen in the pill, so they lowered the amount from 150 micrograms to 50 micrograms. However, in the 1970s it was shown that there was still a risk of clotting; since the dose of oestrogen was now always 50 micrograms, the researchers were able to show that the dose and type of progestogen were the critical factors in making one formulation more risky than another. The companies therefore rushed off to try and lower the dose of progestogen, and to try and improve the progestogens in use.

The early researchers overlooked one important factor: smoking. In the 1960s and 1970s smoking was very fashionable, as its risks had not been appreciated. Taking the pill was also a rather fashionable, avant-garde thing to do (a sign of the 'liberated' woman). So fashion-conscious women were likely to be both taking the pill and smoking, an association which, amazingly, still persists today.

More recent studies have shown that smoking is the single most important risk factor for developing disease of the heart and blood vessels: indeed, women under 50 who smoke are at three times the risk of stroke compared with those who do not smoke. In the initial analysis of the studies which looked at the risk due to the pill, smoking was not taken into account. When the analyses were redone, in the light of the evidence relating to smoking, the risks due to the pill were very much reduced, and, indeed, for non-smokers under the age of 35, disappeared almost completely. In addition, one has to bear in mind that these studies looked at pills which still contained 50 micrograms or more of oestrogen and more progestogen than is used in pills today. Therefore it is reasonable to assume that the risks will be even less for women using low-dose pills.

There are several mechanisms by which the pill can increase the risks of cardiovascular disease, and it is worth having a look at them, even though they are quite complex. Once again, we have to look at the effects of oestrogen and progestogen, and also at what happens when they are combined.

There are two components involved in the development of

disease of the heart and arteries. One is an increased tendency for blood to form clots, blocking off a blood vessel, and therefore starving that part of the body of its food and oxygen. The other is an increased tendency for blood vessels to become 'silted up' and therefore narrowed. Not only does this reduce the amount of blood and therefore food and oxygen reaching that part of the body, but obviously a smaller blood clot than before will be able to totally block the blood vessel, cutting off supplies completely.

The amount of damage which is caused by narrowing of the vessels or clots depends on where the vessels are. The worst places are obviously the heart and the brain. If the arteries leading to the heart become narrowed, the activity of the heart muscle will be reduced. This is what leads to angina. The heart will also have to use more effort to push blood out around the body, so the person's blood pressure will go up. If one or more of those arteries leading to the heart become blocked, part of the heart muscle withers due to lack of oxygen and food, and the person has a heart attack.

Narrowing of the arteries leading to the brain makes a person more likely to develop a clot and therefore cut off vital oxygen and food supplies to that part of the brain. When this happens, the person has a stroke.

Narrowing of arteries is called 'atherosclerosis', and a clot forming in a blood vessel is called a 'thrombosis'. Whereas atherosclerosis seems mostly to happen in and to have its important effects in arteries, thrombosis can occur in both arteries and veins. Arteries bring fresh blood to a part of the body, while veins take the used blood back to the heart to be replenished with oxygen and food, before being pumped out again.

Both oestrogen and progestogens can affect the blood vessels in various ways. Oestrogen tends to increase the tendency of the blood to clot, particularly in veins. It does this by increasing the manufacture of various blood-clotting factors in the blood, though this is partly offset by a simultaneous increase in some of the factors which cause the breakdown of blood clots.

The risk of a venous thrombosis seems to be directly related to the dose of oestrogen in the pill, and is relatively unaffected by either the progestogen or smoking. A venous thrombosis in the calf (called a 'deep vein thrombosis' or DVT) is the most common manifestation of this increase in risk, which is why you should always see your doctor if you get a sudden severe pain and swelling of a calf. The clot itself is not so dangerous, but the real worry is that it may become dislodged and travel onwards.

It may then become trapped in the lungs and cause what is known as a 'pulmonary embolism'. This is a dangerous, though rare condition.

The risk of a venous thrombosis diminishes with decreasing doses of oestrogen, and indeed, studies which have assessed the effect of low-dose pills have found very little increase in the risk at all. Another thing which has been shown in many studies is that the effect of oestrogen on venous thrombosis disappears very rapidly after the pill is stopped, within a couple of weeks in fact.

Arterial disease is much more complicated, and for this we need to look at the effects of oestrogen, progestogens and smoking. Once again, oestrogen has the effect of increasing blood-clotting factors in the blood, though these are to some extent offset by its effect on also increasing the substances which break down blood clots. Smoking comes in here, as it prevents this increase in factors which help break down clots. This means that if you take the pill *and* smoke, your risk of a blood clot in an artery is greater than if you just take the pill or just smoke.

Next we must look at the effects of oestrogen, progestogen and smoking on blood fats. In Chapter 1 we saw that oestrogen increases certain 'good' blood fats, called high-density lipoproteins (HDL), while also decreasing the amount of 'bad' fats, called low-density lipoproteins (LDL). HDL protects against the 'silting up' of arteries (atherosclerosis), whereas LDL tends to cause it. (In fact the situation is much more complicated because there are several kinds of both HDL and LDL, but life, and this book, are much too short to go into that kind of detail.)

Progestogens, on the other hand (apart from the newest ones), tend to lower HDL and raise LDL. This means that while oestrogen is tending to protect you from atherosclerosis, progestogens are trying to cause it.

Smoking also lowers HDL and raises LDL, thus increasing the risk of atherosclerosis. So once again, you can see that whereas in many cases the effects of oestrogen and progestogen will tend to balance each other out, smoking is the crucial extra risk factor. It counteracts the compensatory effects of oestrogen on blood clotting, and adds an extra risk of its own.

In fact, studies have shown that non-smoking women under 35 using low-dose pills have a negligible increase in the risk of arterial disease. Indeed, there is little increase in the risk even up to the age of 45, which is why non-smoking women have been allowed to continue with the pill up to that age for some years now.

However, smokers are at greater risk, and must therefore

stop the pill at the age of 35. By then their risk is greater than that of a 45-year-old non-smoker, so smoking effectively makes your arteries feel 10 years older than they really are.

It should be noted that there are other risk factors for arterial disease, including a family history of a parent or sibling who has had a heart attack or stroke under the age of 45, severe obesity and abnormal levels of blood fats (when not on the pill). A woman who has these risk factors may be at increased risk of arterial disease if she takes the pill, which is why it is important that a full medical and family history are taken before you start the pill. If there are any risk factors, then you should have blood tests to check your blood fats and clotting factors before starting the pill, or while you are on it, to check all is well. In general, this is not considered necessary for women under the age of 35, but becomes more of an issue above that age.

Risk factors are additive, so, for example, if you had a family history of a parent who had a stroke at the age of 40, and you smoke, then you would be at higher risk than if only one of those risk factors were present. This needs to be taken into account when considering a woman's suitability for the pill.

Low-dose pills already seem to give very little risk of arterial disease, but the risks should be reduced even further with the newest pills, containing the new progestogens: desogestrel, gestodene and norgestimate. Unlike the older progestogens, these do not cause a lowering of HDL nor a rise in LDL. On the contrary, some studies have suggested that they actually cause an increase in HDL. Thus, when combined with oestrogen, the resultant effect is as though there were no progestogen there at all, i.e. there should be no bad effects tending to cause arterial disease. This is obviously very reassuring, and has been a major factor influencing the view that these pills could be taken up to the age of 50, provided the woman does not smoke and has no other risk factors for arterial disease. They are also obviously to be preferred for younger women who do have risk factors. The rule of stopping the pill at 35 if you smoke still holds for these pills, however, as smoking is such a strong risk factor in itself.

There has been some publicity suggesting that all women should take these newest pills because even the low-dose but slightly older pills can cause some adverse changes in blood fats. This is taking the argument too far. Many studies have shown that, for young women without risk factors, the older low-dose pills have minimal risks. It is very unlikely that the newest pills would make any real difference to those risks. Indeed, the changes in blood fats which were reported in users of older low-dose pills were still *all within normal limits.* This is something which seems to have been ignored by the media reporting the study.

Having said that, there is bound to be a gradual trend towards the use of the newer pills; after all, why not use something which should be even better than what we had before? But it is important that you realise that there is nothing suddenly wrong with the older pills, just because newer ones are available. They have not suddenly become dangerous, and therefore, if you are perfectly happy on one of them you do not need to go rushing to your doctor to be changed on to a newer one. For the average, healthy, non-smoking woman, the new pills are very unlikely to make any difference to her health risks until she is between the ages of 30 and 35. At that stage, if you intend to continue with the pill, it would be reasonable to change to one of the newer ones. As we will see in Chapter 3, the newer pills often also give fewer of the annoying 'minor' side effects, so you may want to change earlier for that reason, but that should not be allowed to cloud the issue of safety.

The effect of the pill on blood sugar

Blood sugar is often raised in pregnancy, so it is not very surprising that the pill may also have a slight effect. However, the pill does not actually appear to cause diabetes. It may cause a slight rise in blood sugar, particularly in women who have other risk factors for developing diabetes, for example, a family history, a history of diabetes during pregnancy, or severe obesity. Reassuringly, recent studies looking at low-dose pills have shown only very slight changes in blood sugar, which were still within normal levels, and, indeed, low-dose pills can be used even by a woman who is actually diabetic. Changes in blood sugar are thought to be due to progestogen. The newest pills containing the new progestogens have been shown to cause no rise at all in blood sugar, so they would be preferable for women who are diabetic or have risk factors for diabetes.

The pill and surgery

There is often confusion about whether and when to stop the pill before having an operation. The reasoning behind advice to stop the pill before surgery is related to the risk of thrombosis. Anyone who is immobilised for a long time (more than a week), or has a long anaesthetic, is at risk of a deep vein thrombosis regardless of whether or not they take the pill. Thus, it seems reasonable not to add even the tiny increase in risk which may be caused by the pill.

relatively long operations which are likely to make you stay in bed for more than about a week fall into this category. So, for example, simple operations like sterilisation, D & C, or abortions do not give a risk of thrombosis, and it is perfectly all right to continue with the pill right up to the day of the operation, or in the case of an abortion, to start on the day of the operation or the day after.

If you are going to have a bigger operation, it is advisable to stop the pill about four weeks beforehand, and restart about two weeks afterwards. This also applies to surgery on varicose veins: although it is not a major operation, it carries a higher-than-average risk of deep vein thrombosis, so it is best not to take any extra risk, no matter how small. Do not forget to use an alternative method of contraception, however: pregnancy is also associated with an increased risk of thrombosis! Progestogen-only methods, like the Progestogen-Only Pill (see Chapter 5) or injectable progestogens (see Chapter 6), are perfectly safe alternatives to tide you over.

Liver disease

There is a rare form of jaundice which can occur both during pregnancy and on the pill. If due to the pill, it will usually develop within two or three weeks of starting the pill, and will go away when the pill is stopped. It means that the woman will not be able to use the Combined Pill again.

The pill should not be used during any kind of active liver disease, for example infectious hepatitis. However, once tests of liver function have shown a return to normal (which usually takes several months), it is safe to use the pill.

Primary cancer of the liver (i.e. cancer which actually starts in the liver, rather than spreading into it from elsewhere) is extremely rare. Only about one woman in a million develops it in this country. The pill can increase the risk, but it still remains an extremely rare disease.

Hydatidiform mole

This is an unusual condition, in which a pregnancy goes 'out of control' and, instead of developing normally, becomes a tumour, which occasionally turns malignant. It is not caused by the pill, but it is considered unwise for a woman to use the pill while she is under treatment for the condition, since it is influenced by hormonal changes. However, once the hormonal changes associated with it have gone back to normal, it is safe to use the pill. (The hormone which is used as an indicator of what is happening is, in fact, Human Chorionic Gonadotrophin

(HCG), which we discussed in Chapter 1. In this condition, the 'out of control' pregnancy produces huge amounts of HCG, and these can be measured. Once levels of HCG have gone back to normal, i.e. undetectable levels, the condition is considered cured.)

The pill and future fertility

Women are often anxious that taking the pill will decrease their chances of becoming pregnant at a later date. This is not true. Studies have shown that although it may take a few months longer for a woman to become pregnant after stopping the pill, the same number of women will become pregnant in the end, whether or not they took the pill. This is one of the reasons why women on the pill are advised to stop about three months before they would ideally like to become pregnant.

What can happen, however, is that the pill enables women to successfully put off having children until their late thirties. After the age of 30 fertility starts to be reduced quite significantly, so if a woman stops the pill at 36, her chances of becoming pregnant are lower than if she had decided to try for a baby 10 years earlier. Women often forget this, and then blame the pill for their difficulty in becoming pregnant.

Another point is that while a woman is on the pill, her fertility will not be tested. A woman using a barrier method like the cap or sheath is more likely to have an accidental pregnancy at some time, and if so she will know that she is fertile. Also, signs of reduced fertility are likely to be noticed if, for example, she repeatedly takes risks and does not use contraception, but does not become pregnant, or if she stops having periods, and is therefore not ovulating. None of this will be noticeable while a woman takes the pill, because it removes the normal menstrual cycle altogether, and is so effective at preventing pregnancy. Once again, the woman may blame the pill when she stops and finds it difficult to become pregnant, but all that has happened is that the pill masked a problem which was there anyway.

The term 'post-pill amenorrhoea' is yet another example of this phenomenon. Sometimes, when a woman stops taking the pill, it takes more than six months for her periods to return. In fact, about 2 per cent of women stop having periods for six months or more when they are not on the pill. However, if they had this tendency, it would have been masked while they were on the pill. Once again, although the pill is not the cause, it gets the blame because the problem is only noticed after the pill has stopped being taken.

Accidental pregnancy while taking the pill
Women are often worried about what would happen to a baby if they did become pregnant while taking the pill. Indeed, some women are worried about whether their baby might be abnormal even if they had stopped the pill, but became pregnant shortly afterwards.

On the latter point, the evidence all shows there is no increase in the risk of miscarriage or of an abnormal baby. Nor is there any tendency for an increased likelihood of male or female babies.

The evidence is also reassuring for women who conceive while actually still taking the pill. However, it must be said that because this is such a rare event, there is correspondingly less evidence available. About 2 per cent of all babies born are abnormal, and there does not appear to be any increase among babies of women who conceive on the pill. Obviously, if you find you are pregnant, you should stop taking the pill, but there does not seem to be any reason to worry about the effects on the baby.

Cancer of the cervix
Cancer of the cervix is on the increase, particularly in young women. A great deal of research has focused on this cancer during the last 20 years, but there is still much we do not know about what causes it or how to prevent it. The only definite causal factor is sex: to all intents and purposes, if you don't ever have sex, you won't get cervical cancer. This is not a practical proposition for most women, and certainly would take family planning to a new extreme.

Sex and sexual behaviour are extremely complicated topics. At first it was thought that it was quite simple: the earlier a woman starts to have sex, and the more men she has sex with, the more likely she is to get cervical cancer. Then women turned up with cervical cancer who had only ever had sex with one man. Why should they have developed cancer? In this way, the concept of the 'high-risk male' was discovered. Basically it means that the more women a man has sex with, the more likely those women are to get cervical cancer. So it is not just the number of sexual partners a woman has, the number of partners men have is just as important.

What is it about sex which is so dangerous? Unfortunately, we still do not know. Various things have been suggested, from sperm, to bacteria, to viruses. At present, the most likely candidate seems to be the genital wart or human papillomavirus (HPV). However, it certainly does not produce cancer on its own. HPV infection seems to be so common that I would not be surprised to find it in my sandwiches at lunchtime! If it was the only important factor, there would be no women left. In animals, when a papillomavirus causes cancer it always needs help from something else. For example, bovine papillomavirus can cause stomach cancer in cows, but only if they eat bracken as well. There is more and more evidence suggesting that in women, this help may come from smoking.

Just as the early pill studies did not take smoking into account when looking at the risks of arterial disease, neither did they look at smoking in relation to cervical cancer. This is a major problem since, as I have mentioned before, pill users are known to be more likely to smoke than non-users. In addition, pill users were not likely to be using sheaths, which are known to protect against cervical cancer, presumably because they help prevent the transmission of sexually acquired diseases. If there is any effect of semen or sperm (this is just conjecture, as there is no proof of such an effect), then obviously pill users will again be at greater risk compared with users of barrier methods, since the cervix of a woman on the pill is still exposed to semen. Also studies have shown that women who smoke are more likely to be having sex more often than women who do not smoke, and women on the pill are also likely to be having sex more often than non-users. There have also been studies showing that women who use the pill tend to have more sexual partners than non-users.

There is not a single study which has even attempted to try and unravel all of these entangled risk factors. As you can see, the pill is intimately related to sexual behaviour and to smoking habits, so it is very difficult to separate their effects from the effect of the pill itself. This is why studies which implicate the pill as a risk factor for cervical cancer should be viewed with caution, and certainly the effect of smoking is much stronger. I cannot foresee that any study will be able to set up a control group for comparison for every single other possibility. For instance, just imagine trying to find out how many partners each of the men in a particular woman's life had had in the past, or asking people how often they had had sex during the last 10 years.

So although the pill is implicated as a weak risk factor in some studies, the evidence is not strong enough to make a real case. You would definitely do your cervix a much bigger favour by giving up smoking. And, as for all women, regular cervical smears (at least every three years) will catch changes in the cells of the cervix before they can develop into cancer, regardless of whatever made those cells start to change abnormally in the first place. Although we still do not really know what causes cervical cancer, at least we do have a means of preventing it.

Breast cancer

It would be quite easy to write a whole book just on this subject. The relationship between the pill and breast cancer is very interesting, not least because of its many contradictions. As I mentioned earlier, breast cancer appears, to a great extent, to have the same risk factors as both ovarian and endometrial cancer. They are all associated with early onset of periods, late menopause and having no children. In addition, breast cancer appears in some studies to be less common in women who breastfeed for a long time. What do all these factors have in common? Periods, and therefore ovulation. It appears that the more periods, and therefore the more times you ovulate in your life, the higher your chances of developing cancers of the breast, ovary and endometrium (lining of the womb). Women who breastfeed for a long time often do not have periods until they stop, so that reduces the number of times they ovulate. And the pill is known to give considerable protection against cancer of the ovary and cancer of the endometrium, presumably because it prevents ovulation. Not only that, but, as we have seen, it strongly protects a woman from developing benign (non-cancerous) breast disease. So, in theory, you would think that everything is in favour of the pill also being protective against breast cancer. And yet studies have not shown this to be the case. On the contrary, the majority of 'pill scares' since the early 1980s have been due to studies which actually suggested an *increased* risk of breast cancer due to the pill.

Unfortunately, we still have little idea of what causes breast cancer. A Western diet (high in saturated fats, i.e. dairy products and red meat) has been strongly associated with an increased risk of breast cancer, but there is no proof that it can actually cause it. It is certainly very striking that women who live in the developing world have a much lower risk of breast cancer. The most interesting finding relating to the diet theory is that Japanese women living in Japan and eating a diet which is low in saturated fat have a very low incidence of breast cancer. However, when these women emigrate to the United States, and presumably start eating junk food, their risk of breast cancer goes up dramatically.

Another feature of breast cancer, in which it seems to differ from ovarian and endometrial cancers, is that it is quite definitely familial. If a woman's mother or sister has breast cancer, she is at increased risk of developing it herself.

However, one reassuring aspect of the studies so far is that the pill does not appear to add to the risk which is already there, i.e. women with a family history of breast cancer are at increased risk, but it does not seem that the pill actually adds to this risk.

There may well be other risk factors for breast cancer which we have not yet discovered, and this obviously makes it more difficult to draw firm conclusions about any aspect of the disease.

Whenever you hear about a study looking at the relationship between the pill and breast cancer, you should remember that the women in these studies were likely to be taking high-dose pills which are no longer used today. Despite this, a vast weight of evidence suggests that there is no increased risk of breast cancer due to the pill after the age of 25. There are very large and well-conducted studies which support this view. At present, the controversy is all about pill use before the age of 25.

It all started in 1983 when an American study was published which suggested an increase in risk with pill use below the age of 25. This study was looking specifically at breast cancer which developed before the age of 36. The researchers tried to link the risk with different kinds of progestogens, but this was later shown to be invalid.

In May 1989 a similar study was published, this time in the UK. Once again, the study looked at women in whom breast cancer developed below the age of 36. This study was more interesting because it actually looked at some women who had used low-dose pills, and gave the risks for those. Overall, the researchers found a relative risk of 1.43 for four to eight years' use, and of 1.74 for more than eight years' use below the age of 25. (The concept of relative risk is actually quite simple: a relative risk of 1 means that there is no effect of the pill, i.e. the risk is the same for users and non-users. A relative risk of less than 1 means that the effect of the pill is to protect against breast cancer. A relative risk of more than one means that the pill increases the risk. So, for example, a relative risk of 2 means that pill users have twice the risk compared with non-users, while a relative risk of 1.74 means they have roughly one and three quarter times the risk of non-users.)

The vast majority of the increase in risk was actually concentrated in the group of women who had used high-dose pills. Figure 2.1 shows the results for low-dose pills. The researchers were only able to analyse the results for some brands, which were taken by reasonably large numbers of women, and none of the pills containing the new progestogens could be included, since they were not yet available when the study was done (it finished in 1983).

You will notice that there is little or no increase in risk for these pills, and indeed, one brand (Logynon/Trinordiol) appears to be protective! This may well be an artefact, due to the relatively small numbers of women using this pill, as may be the apparent very slight increase in risk in women using the Ovysmen/Brevinor brand. It is probably best to go by the other two brands which had by far the greatest number of women months of use. You will see that for these, the risk was not altered either way (a 0.08 difference is not significant). The results of this study are therefore reassuring for women currently using, or thinking of using, the modern low-dose pills.

Figure 2.1 Relative risks of breast cancer for low-dose pills.
(Source: UK National Case Control Study, *Lancet*, 6 May 1989)

Brand	Ostrogen (mcg)	Progestogen (mcg)	Total woman months of use	Relative risk
Brevinor/ Ovysmen	35	500 norethisterone	711	1.18
Logynon/ Trinordiol	32	90 levonorgestrel	1490	0.83
Eugynon 30/ Ovran 30	30	250 levonorgestrel	14941	1.00
Microgynon/ Ovranette	30	150 levonorgestrel	15348	1.08

Indeed, we have reason to be even more optimistic about the newest pills, containing the new progestogens. The reason is their effect on Sex Hormone Binding Globulin (SHBG), which I mentioned in Chapter 1. You may remember that the older progestogens have the effect of lowering the amount of SHBG in the blood. Interestingly, this has also been noticed in women who have breast cancer, i.e. they have been found to have lower levels of SHBG than women who are healthy. The new progestogens do not lower the SHBG level, indeed they actually raise it, so they are acting in the opposite way to what happens in breast cancer. Some doctors have actually suggested that these new pills may be protective against breast cancer: I feel that it is premature to make such claims when we have absolutely no evidence to back it up. However, I think it is reasonable to hope that, in view of this effect on SHBG and the fact that even the older low-dose pills do not appear to increase the risk, these new pills are even less likely to increase the risk of breast cancer.

There is an interesting theory which has been put forward to try and explain why young women taking the pill may appear to have an increased risk of breast cancer, while older women do not. Indeed, some studies have suggested that in older women, the pill may actually have a protective effect, and also that it seems to slow down the growth of breast cancer which has developed. The theory is this: young women very commonly have lumpy, tender breasts, but breast cancer is extremely rare under the age of 35. A young woman who goes to her doctor with a breast lump is likely to be dismissed, partly because it may be difficult to distinguish between the particular lump which is worrying her, compared with the rest of her lumpy breast, and partly because the doctor knows her chances of having cancer are very low. Thus, if she really has a cancer, she is less likely to notice it herself because of the general lumpiness, and also her doctor is less likely to diagnose it, so she will be more likely to be diagnosed a few years later, when it has grown in size and become unmistakable.

A young woman on the pill, however, is much less likely to have lumpy breasts, because the pill is so good at preventing this. So, not only is she more likely to notice a suspicious lump, but it will also be easier for her doctor to diagnose. Thus, a woman on the pill is likely to have her breast cancer picked up sooner and therefore when she is younger than a woman who is not on the pill. This might explain an apparent increase in risk for young women developing breast cancer while taking the pill. This is only a theory, however, and the question remains unresolved.

It does seem strange that pill use only appears to cause an increased risk in women under 25, and that breast cancer differs so much in this respect when compared with ovarian and endometrial cancers. There is another interesting idea which has been put forward to explain this. When the pill causes the ovaries to 'shut down', both they and the uterus really do cease to function in the way they normally would, i.e. the ovaries do not produce hormones or eggs, and the lining of the uterus becomes much thinner and stops its normal 'preparations' for a possible pregnancy. However, although the pill does make the breasts less active, in that there is a marked reduction in benign breast lumps, they can still respond to the synthetic hormone, often in a similar way to natural oestrogen. So the 'shutting down' effect is actually much weaker than in the uterus and ovaries.

Also, it has been noticed that although, in the long term, having a child, particularly when young, gives protection against breast cancer, in the short term (for three or four years afterwards), the woman is actually at *greater* risk. It is possible that the short-term increase in the level of hormones during pregnancy tends to give a favourable environment for breast cancer to develop. Similarly, if the pill is taken by a young woman, the hormones may temporarily increase the risk of breast cancer, and then the risk disappears after a few years. Once again, these are only theories, and we need evidence to back them up. Research continues, and the results of studies in the next few years may tell us more about the pills we are really interested in, namely low-dose pills. Unfortunately, it will be many years before any hard evidence emerges about the newest pills, since they only started to be introduced in about 1984.

RISKS VERSUS BENEFITS

As a final point, I would like to mention the latest results of an ongoing study, which were published in December 1989. This study has been following a large group of women, some of whom use the pill, while others use different methods of family planning. The study began in 1968, and recruited over 17,000 women, so it is large and has been going on for over 20 years.

The researchers looked at the causes of death in these women, and compared pill users with non-users. Overall, they found that the pill users were actually slightly *less* likely to have died, compared to non-users – the relative risk for pill users was 0.9. Much of this low risk was due to the large, protective effect of the pill against ovarian and endometrial cancers, a benefit which easily outweighs all the other possible health risks. And this in women who, for the majority of the study, would have been taking high-dose pills. It is certainly a reassuring result.

However, each woman is different, and therefore each woman will need to make up her own mind about the risk:benefit ratio in her own individual case. Your doctor should be able to help answer any questions you may have, or, for more detailed information, I would recommend John Guillebaud's book *The Pill* (see Further Reading).

3

WHICH PILL SHOULD I TAKE? – DEALING WITH SIDE EFFECTS

This chapter looks at the so-called 'minor' side effects of the pill, which are not at all 'minor' to the women experiencing them!

Many of these types of side effects can be explained by looking at the balance of oestrogen and progestogen in a particular pill formulation. In Chapter 1 we saw that oestrogen and progestogen each have their own specific effects in the body, although these are modified when the two are combined in the pill. The actual effect a woman experiences from any given brand will depend on which of the two hormones is having the most noticeable effect.

Women often cannot understand why their friends are happy on a brand which did not suit them. Conversely, I am often asked why someone a woman knows was given a different pill to the one I am suggesting for her. There are several factors to be taken into account.

First of all, no two women are alike, and therefore the way they react to the pill will not necessarily be the same. Each woman has her own personal hormonal balance, and although her own hormone production will be essentially stopped by the pill, a little still goes on, and the amount of each hormone will be specific to her body. So, if you like, each woman's body is already used to either an 'oestrogen dominance' or a 'progestogen dominance' of her own.

If a woman whose body is used to being 'progestogen-dominant' is given an 'oestrogen-dominant' pill, several things may happen. She may develop breast tenderness in response to the oestrogen bias, which may or may not improve with time. She

Figure 3.1 List of oestrogenic and progestogenic side effects.

Ostrogenic	Progestogenic *(but not caused, or very much less, by the new progestogens: desogestrel, gestodene, norgestimate)*
Breast enlargement	Acne
Breast tenderness	Greasy hair
Bloating	Hirsutism (excess hair)
Weight gain due to water retention	Weight gain due to increased appetite
Nausea	Depression
Non-infective vaginal discharge	Loss of libido
Some headaches	Vaginal dryness
Chloasma (brown patches on the face)	
Photosensitivity	

may experience feelings of bloating. On the other hand, she may be delighted because her acne has improved, her hair is less greasy and she has more interest in sex. Or she may have a combination of desirable and undesirable effects.

If a woman whose body is used to being 'oestrogen-dominant' is given a 'progestogen-dominant' pill, once again she may experience various effects. She may be delighted that her breasts are less tender and she seems to have fewer headaches, but gaze in horror at her complexion, which used to be so clear and is now covered in nasty spots.

Often all that is needed is time for the body to achieve a new sense of balance, and then such side effects improve. Three months is about the length of time you should allow to see if there is an improvement.

Changing pills can have the same effect at first. If you are changed from a relatively 'oestrogen-dominant' pill to a relatively 'progestogen-dominant' one, or vice versa, you may well get some side effects during the first month or two.

So, when starting the pill for the first time (or after a long break), it is useful to take into account your own characteristics. Do you tend to have acne or greasy hair? Then an 'oestrogen-dominant' pill should improve things, though you may pay the price of some breast tenderness at first. On the other hand, do you often have tender breasts? In that case you should be happier on a 'progestogen-dominant' pill.

Sometimes your medical history needs to be taken into account. For example, women with a history of benign (non-cancerous) breast lumps, endometriosis or fibroids are best off with a 'progestogen-dominant' pill.

Each woman's history and characteristics are different, so she may well not be given the same pill as her best friend.

If you have been on the pill before, your experiences in the past will act as guidance. This is why it is very important to try and remember which pills you have taken and whether they suited you. Obviously, if you have had side effects on a particular type of pill, it would be best to try a different one next time.

Another major factor is that it has been shown that there is a tenfold variation in the absorption of the pill by different women. This means that if you give 10 women the same pill at the same time of day, they will each have different blood levels of the hormones when you measure them later. Obviously, this means they will experience different side effects, even though they are taking exactly the same pill. For example, the woman who has the highest blood levels may find she is better suited to a lower dose pill, while the woman who has the lowest levels may need a higher dose pill. These two women will then presumably have similar blood levels, but will in fact be taking different strength pills. Things are rarely as they first seem.

A third factor is doctor variability, and even intra-doctor variability! Different doctors have their own 'favourite' pills with which they are most familiar. You must remember that there is such a large choice of pills that doctors who do not specialise in family planning are unlikely to be really familiar with the effects of each one. Not only do different doctors have their own favourites, but that favourite may change over time. This may be because a newer, better pill becomes available, or because the doctor realises, through experience, that a different pill gives fewer problems.

YOUR FIRST TIME ON THE PILL

To be honest, within limits it matters little which pill you are first given if you are young, a non-smoker and healthy. You should however check that the pill you have been given does not contain more than 35 micrograms of oestrogen (unless there is a specific reason, such as an interacting drug; see Chapter 4). Nowadays, I would say that if you are starting the pill, you might as well start on one of the newest pills,

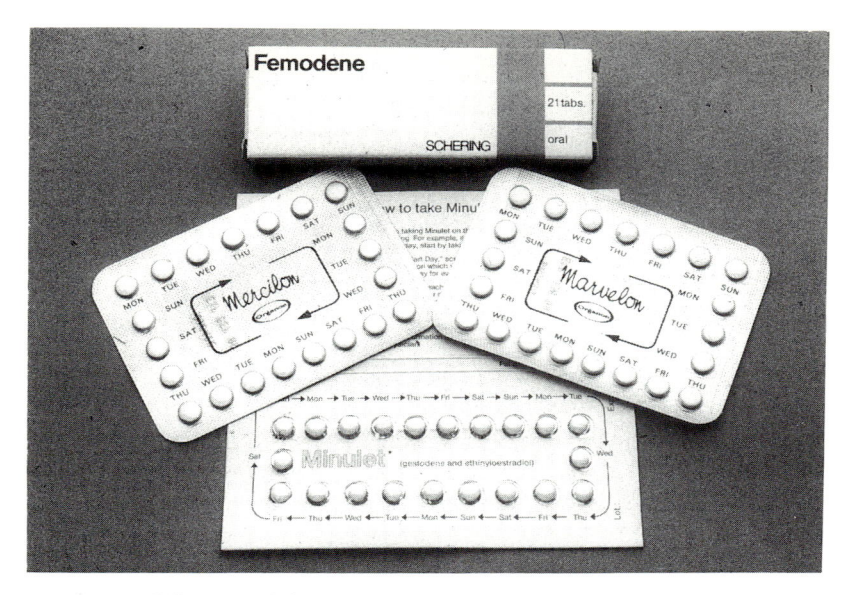

Figure 3.2 Pills containing new progestogens.

containing the new progestogens. This means starting on Marvelon, Minulet/Femodene or Mercilon.

As you can see, Marvelon and Minulet/Femodene (Minulet and Femodene are identical, just made by different companies) contain 30 micrograms of oestrogen, combined with different progestogens. Don't worry about the dose of progestogen as it isn't comparable. In fact, the 75 micrograms of gestodene in Minulet/Femodene are actually rather stronger than the 300 micrograms of desogestrel in Marvelon.

Mercilon has only 20 micrograms of oestrogen, combined with the same amount and type of progestogen as Marvelon.

Figure 3.3 Formulations of the new pills

Minulet/Femodene	30 mcg ethinyloestradiol (oestrogen) + 75 mcg gestodene
Marvelon	30 mcg ethinyloestradiol + 150 mcg desogestrel
Mercilon	20 mcg ethinyloestradiol + 150 mcg desogestrel

You may ask, why not start with Mercilon, since it is a lower dose?

In fact, I do not routinely recommended this, for the following reasons. Many women, if not most, have side effects when they first start the pill. These are usually nausea, some headaches, odd aches and pains and feeling a little bloated. If you think about it, these are very similar to the problems women often have in early pregnancy – not that surprising, since the pill works by making the brain think the woman is pregnant. In pregnancy, these problems usually settle down after the first two or three months, and the same is true for the pill. However, some women suffer badly during the first couple of months, and it does not seem to make any difference whether they started off with 20 micrograms of oestrogen or 30: it is the adaptation process to being on the pill which is the critical factor. In addition, being on the pill for the first time is often nerve-racking, as you don't know what to expect, but you fear the worst. Every time you have a headache, you wonder, 'Is it due to the pill?' All this anxiety does not help your tolerance.

If you have been feeling really rough for the last two months, and you go and see a doctor, who merely says, 'There, there, it will get better in another few months, keep taking the tablets,' how will you feel? Frustrated, depressed and ready to give up the pill altogether? The very sight of the packet each morning is now making you feel ill. This is not silly. I once worked in a cancer unit, where I had to give patients chemotherapy (very strong anti-cancer drugs). These drugs had awful side effects and, in particular, they made people very sick. Patients who had to have them for long periods of time often reached the stage where they would actually start to vomit when they saw me walking down the ward in their direction. I can tell you, this did nothing for my confidence as a young doctor, nor for my self-esteem! The same type of thing can happen in any situation where you begin to associate something – like a blue pill packet, for example – with feeling ill. Although it is true you may well get better in another couple of months, psychologically, you want a change to something different, and preferably now.

This is where the pink pill packet comes in! Not only does Mercilon have slightly less oestrogen, but it looks different as well. Changing 'downwards' in this way usually helps women with teething problems quite rapidly. You feel better, quickly, and are reassured both physically and psychologically.

If you had started off with Mercilon, you might well be feeling the same as on a 30-microgram pill, but what are you going to do? Change *upwards* to Marvelon? There is no lower-dose option available. So then you have to stick it out.

You may ask, 'But what about those women who are put on a 30-microgram pill and feel fine on it? Aren't they being put at risk by staying on a higher dose?' The answer is that there is no evidence that Mercilon is actually any 'safer' in the long term than Marvelon. Their effects on blood fats, sugars and clotting factors are very similar. It may be that a 'ceiling' has been reached and that even if you lower the dose, you make no further difference to the health risks (which by now are extremely small). In addition, many women are very happy on a slightly more 'oestrogenic' pill, which gives them a wonderful complexion. And if, of course, they develop side effects at any time, they can always then change to Mercilon. I tend to recommend changing to Mercilon to women over 40 who wish to stay on the pill, simply because it seems reasonable to give them the lowest dose possible, even without any real supporting evidence (this is called making the doctor feel happier!).

Whichever pill you start with, you need to give it at least two months, and preferably three, to know whether it is going to suit you. Then, if you are not happy, your next pill can be chosen to correct the particular side effects you are experiencing. Let us look at the common ones first.

BREAKTHROUGH BLEEDING

This means bleeding other than during the pill-free week, when you have your 'period'. Sometimes it can be heavy, sometimes just spotting. Many women seem to get particularly worried when they see what looks like dark, old blood. This is quite meaningless and does not have any sinister implications.

What causes breakthrough bleeding?

Usually what it means is that the level of hormones present in your blood is not high enough to keep the endometrium (lining of the womb) firmly under control. It does not, however, mean that you are at risk of pregnancy. The hormone levels required to keep the endometrium 'quiet' are higher than those needed to prevent ovulation, so even if you have breakthrough bleeding, there is enough hormone there to prevent pregnancy. What it does mean, however, is that you don't have much of a safety net. So if you were to then go and forget pills, or take interacting medicines, you might well be at risk of pregnancy.

Why are your hormone levels not high enough? Well, the most obvious explanation is that your pill is not strong enough for you. As we have seen, there is a tenfold variation in blood levels between different women, which means that in some women either less is going in (i.e. being absorbed from the gut) or more is going out (i.e. being destroyed in the liver). Less absorption may occur if you have a stomach upset, or if you take broad spectrum antibiotics like penicillin or tetracycline. This is discussed in detail in the next chapter. It occurs because certain bacteria in the gut help to increase the amount of oestrogen which is absorbed. Broad spectrum antibiotics are designed to kill as many bacteria as possible, and they don't discriminate between good ones and bad ones. So these helpful bacteria disappear along with the rest. Interestingly, vegetarians also seem to have fewer of these bacteria, so they sometimes need a stronger pill to give adequate blood levels.

If you have a stomach upset or are taking a course of antibiotics, you need to use additional contraceptive precautions. Full instructions for this are given in Chapter 4. In such cases, the breakthrough bleeding will stop when you are better or have finished the antibiotics.

Another common cause of less hormone being absorbed is that the woman has forgotten to take one or more pills. In this case, the breakthrough bleeding often occurs several days, even a week after the missed pill. Just one forgotten pill can lead to a week of breakthrough bleeding. You must remember that the dose of hormones nowadays is so low that it does not give you much room for error. When high-dose pills were being used, women could forget several pills without either bleeding or becoming pregnant – but at the cost of side effects and health risks. Making an effort to remember is surely preferable. What to do if you miss a pill is discussed fully in Chapter 4.

Breakthrough bleeding is not uncommon when you first start a new pill. In general, unless it really is unbearable, you should wait a couple of months and see if it settles down. If it does not, and you can find no obvious reason why you are absorbing too little hormone, then the chances are that your liver is getting rid of it rather fast.

The enzymes in the liver which destroy the pill work at different rates in different people. It is not possible to tell in advance which women have fast enzymes and which have slow ones. Neither is abnormal. However, a woman who has fast enzymes will need to take more hormone to achieve the same blood level as a woman who has slow enzymes. So she will need a higher-dose pill. Of course, although it is a higher dose, this does not mean she will suffer more side effects or health risks. The amount her body can actually use is the same as for another woman who is on a lower-dose pill but has slower enzymes.

Artificial speeding up of the liver enzymes can occur as a result of certain medicines, particularly those used in the treatment of epilepsy and tuberculosis. If this applies to you, you will need to be on a higher-dose pill. This is discussed fully in Chapter 4.

There is another way in which breakthrough bleeding can occur, which is by temporarily *increasing* the absorption of oestrogen from the stomach. This can happen if you decide to be extra healthy for a while and start taking large doses (over 400 mg) of vitamin C. Vitamin C actually increases the absorption of oestrogen, and therefore converts your low-dose pill into a higher-dose pill. This is fine until you forget to take it, or decide to stop, and after all few people are really meticulous about taking a vitamin every single day. The effect is then similar to that of missing a pill, because your body suddenly receives less oestrogen than before. Result: breakthrough bleeding. If you do want to take vitamin C supplements while you are on the pill, it is best to take less than 400 mg per day (which in any case is far more than the body needs) and also to try not to take it at the same time as your pill. If you can leave a gap of more than four hours between the two, you should not have any problems, since by then one will have been fully absorbed before the other gets there, so to speak.

A similar effect to that of vitamin C can occur with the antibiotic Septrin (Cotrimoxazole), though by a different mechanism. This antibiotic (which is often used to treat cystitis) slows down the liver enzymes, thereby permitting more hormone to enter the system. Once again, you may find you get breakthrough bleeding when you stop, though this will not place you at risk of pregnancy. In this case, taking the tablets at different times will not help.

If there is no obvious reason why you are getting breakthrough bleeding, and it persists even after a change of pill, your doctor should examine you to check that there is no other reason why you are bleeding. Although this is unlikely, one should always bear in mind things like infections or other gynaecological conditions.

So, if you do get breakthrough bleeding, and it appears that the solution lies in changing your pill, which one should you take? This depends, of course, on which pill you are currently taking. Here are a few guidelines, though of course I cannot really cover every possibility. In general, the first thing to do is to increase the strength of the progestogen, keeping the oestrogen dose the same. If that does not work, then the dose of oestrogen should also be increased. You should give each change of pill two or three months to see if the problem has been solved. Remember that as long as you get breakthrough bleeding (BTB), the pill is not strong enough for you, so it is perfectly safe to increase the dose.

If your breakthrough bleeding occurs regularly in the first week of your packet, it may help to shorten the pill-free week, perhaps to four days instead of seven. If in the pill-free week your hormone levels drop to below the level at which bleeding can be controlled, it should help to try and build up the hormone level again more quickly, by restarting sooner.

Here are some hints on dealing with BTB for specific pill formulations (see also the flow chart on the next page).

BTB on Mercilon or Marvelon (there is not enough difference between them to warrant changing from Mercilon to Marvelon): change to Minulet/Femodene. If this still does not work, change to two tablets of Mercilon per day (this increases the oestrogen dose to 40 micrograms). If this is still not enough, you can take one Marvelon plus one Mercilon per day, thereby increasing the oestrogen dose to 50 micrograms. There are, in fact, some 50 microgram pills available, which would mean you need only take one a day, but none contain the new progestogens, so it seems reasonable to try and still have the benefit by doubling up on the lower-dose pills. You can go on increasing the dose until you no longer get breakthrough bleeding.

BTB on Ovysmen/Brevinor (which contain 35 micrograms of oestrogen, plus 500 micrograms of norethisterone): BTB on this formulation is so common that it is almost more surprising if you don't have it. Equally common is to miss withdrawal bleeds, especially if you have had BTB. This pill suffers from being so oestrogenically biased as to be ridiculous (good for skin, but breast tenderness is another common problem). A change to Marvelon is usually enough, and if that doesn't work, follow the rules for BTB on Marvelon.

BTB on Microgynon/Ovranette (which contains 30 micrograms of oestrogen plus 150 micrograms of levonorgestrel): this is unusual, but if it occurs, try Minulet/Femodene first. If that doesn't work, move to the two tablets of Mercilon approach.

BTB on triphasic pills (Trinordiol/Logynon/Logynon ED, Trinovum/Trinovum ED): try Minulet/Femodene and so on.

BTB on Neocon (35 micrograms of oestrogen plus 1 milligram of norethisterone acetate) or Loestrin 30 (30 micrograms of oestrogen plus 1.5 milligrams of norethisterone acetate): if this occurs, Minulet/Femodene is a possibility, but cannot be

Figure 3.4 Flow chart showing ways of changing pill if breakthrough bleeding occurs.

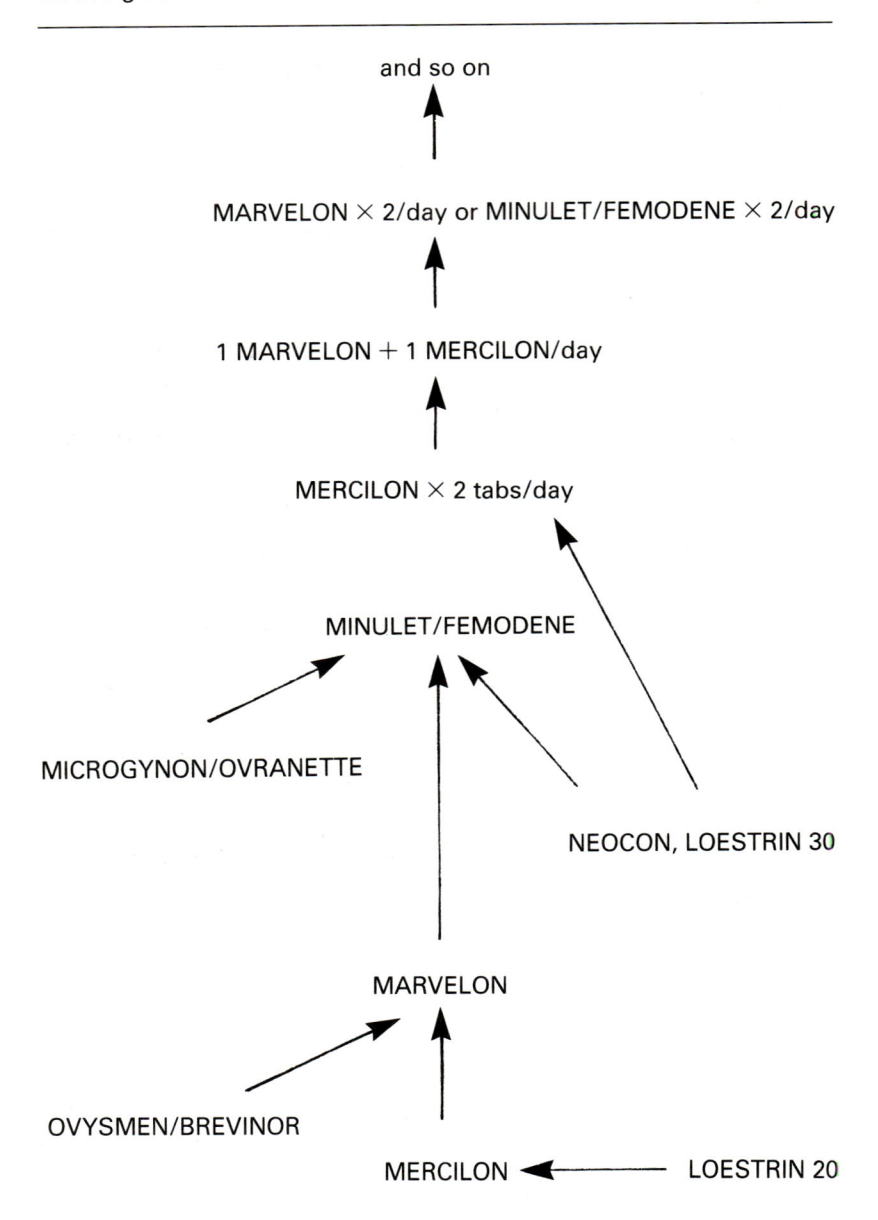

and so on
↑
MARVELON × 2/day or MINULET/FEMODENE × 2/day
↑
1 MARVELON + 1 MERCILON/day
↑
MERCILON × 2 tabs/day
↑
MINULET/FEMODENE
↑
MICROGYNON/OVRANETTE ↗   ↖ NEOCON, LOESTRIN 30

MARVELON
↑
OVYSMEN/BREVINOR ↗

MERCILON ← LOESTRIN 20

Figure 3.5 Oestrogen-dominant and progestogen-dominant pills.

A. 'Older pills' (in descending order of 'strength' of the effect)

Oestrogen-dominant

Ovysmen/Brevinor
35 mcg ethinyloestradiol +
ethinyloestradiol
500 mg norethisterone

Neocon/Norimin
35 mcg ethinyloestradiol
+ 1 mg norethisterone

Progestogen-dominant

Loestrin 30
30 mcg ethinyloestradiol
+ 1.5 mg norethisterone

Microgynon/Ovranette
30 mcg ethinyloestradiol
+ 150 mcg levonorgestrel

Loestrin 20
20 mcg ethinyloestradiol
+ 1 mg norethisterone acetate

B. Triphasics: effect varies according to phase of cycle, therefore cannot be properly placed in such a classification

Trinovum
21 tablets of 35 mcg ethinyloestradiol + 500 mcg, 700 mcg and 1 mg

norethisterone (7 tablets of each)

Trinordiol/Logynon
6 tablets containing 30 mcg ethinyloestradiol
+
50 mcg levonorgestrel, 5 tablets containing 40 mcg ethinyloestradiol + 75 mcg levonorgestrel, 10 tablets containing 30 mcg ethinyloestradiol + 125 mcg levonorgestrel

C. Newest pills: none exhibit real progestogenic side effects, but vary in their 'oestrogen dominance' and control of bleeding

'Oestrogen dominance'

Marvelon (most)

Minulet/Femodene

Mercilon

Cycle control

Minulet/Femodene (best cycle control)

Marvelon and Mercilon

---

guaranteed to be strong enough. If you have had a very bad time with the bleeding, I would suggest going straight on to the two Mercilons per day stage.

BTB on Loestrin 20 (20 micrograms of oestrogen plus 1 milligram of norethisterone acetate): this is almost universal, which is why this pill has never been very popular. A change to Mercilon will probably be enough, or you can work up from there.

I realise that Mercilon and Minulet/Femodene may not yet be available everywhere, though Marvelon is now widely used. If this is the case, here are some general guidelines.

BTB on Marvelon will often resolve itself with Microgynon/Ovranette. If not try either Loestrin 30 or Neocon. Pills containing 50 micrograms of oestrogen are available, and you may need to use one of these if the BTB persists.

MISSED WITHDRAWAL BLEEDS

Contrary to what most women think, it is very unlikely that this is due to pregnancy. Indeed, you can quite easily have withdrawal bleeds while you are pregnant. The most likely cause is simply that not enough lining built up in the womb and so there is nothing to come away. Blood does not 'build up inside'. Having said that, if you have normally had withdrawal bleeds on a particular brand, it is worth having a pregnancy test just to be sure. If you had breakthrough bleeding during the last packet, you may well not have a withdrawal bleed afterwards, since what lining there was has already been shed. In that case, the chances are you will have a withdrawal bleed after your next packet (assuming you do not have breakthrough bleeding again).

Missing withdrawal bleeds is not dangerous and, indeed, has many advantages, the most obvious one being that you do not have the bother of bleeding, despite being able to have your normal pill-free week. Trying to induce withdrawal bleeds by changing brands is a rather hit-and-miss affair. A more 'progestogen-dominant' pill may help, but there is no guarantee. It is often just a case of 'try it and see'. Unless it really upsets you, I would recommend doing nothing and getting used to the idea instead.

BREAST TENDERNESS/ENLARGEMENT

This is quite common when a woman first starts taking the pill, but should settle within the first two or three months. If it does not, a change should help. Breast tenderness and enlargement are oestrogenic side effects, so a change to a more 'progestogen-dominant' pill should help.

Breast tenderness is particularly common on Ovysmen/Brevinor, and may resolve itself just by changing to Marvelon. However, Marvelon itself is quite 'oestrogenic' so that may not be enough. Minulet/Femodene may do the trick, or if that is not available, Microgynon/Ovranette. Another option is to simply reduce the dose of oestrogen by changing to Mercilon (but not Loestrin 20 if possible, because you are then very likely to have BTB).

Breast tenderness in the last week of a triphasic pill will often improve if you change to a monophasic pill (i.e. one which has the same dose of hormones all month). Obviously do not choose one which itself often causes breast tenderness!

If none of these pill changes help, and you want to stay on the pill if possible, you may want to consider looking at your diet. It does seem that if you eat a lot of saturated fats (found in dairy products and red meat) you are more likely to have breast tenderness. You should try and cut down on these, and, if you do eat dairy produce, try to use low-fat versions of milk, cheese and yoghurt. Evening Primrose Oil is a mixture of polyunsaturated fats, and may give extra benefit if you are already cutting down on saturated fats.

Some women also find Vitamin B6 helpful, usually in doses of around 50 mg per day.

It is unusual for breast tenderness to be 'incurable' on the pill. However, if this does seem to be the case, you may need to stop the Combined Pill and perhaps try the Progestogen-Only Pill (see Chapter 5) or an injectable progestogen (see Chapter 6).

MILKY DISCHARGE FROM THE NIPPLES

The pill can cause a harmless increase in the production of the hormone prolactin, which stimulates milk production in the breasts. However, if you get a milky discharge from the nipples, you should not assume it is harmless and ignore it. There is an extremely rare tumour of the pituitary gland which can also lead to a large increase in the production of prolactin. This type of tumour does not spread to other parts of the body, but is very nasty, because it can cause problems in the brain just due to its size. In particular, it can lead to blindness, so you should always see a doctor, and he or she will send off a blood sample to check your prolactin level. You may also have a skull X-ray, as the tumour can sometimes be detected in this way. If you do turn out to have a pituitary tumour, you will need specialist treatment and monitoring (though the treatment itself usually just involves taking a medicine called bromocriptine to shrink the tumour). It used to be thought that the pill could cause this type of tumour or make it worse, but this is no longer true for the modern low-dose pills. In fact, nowadays it is quite possible that the specialist endocrinologist will allow you to carry on taking the pill, even while you are under treatment.

BLOATING/WATER RETENTION

This is an oestrogenic effect, so in general, the thing to do is to reduce the dose of oestrogen and/or use a more 'progestogen-dominant' pill. One way in which this very occasionally shows itself is called the carpal tunnel syndrome. This is more common in pregnancy, and is due to the water retention which occurs then. Swelling of the wrists causes pressure on a nerve which has to pass through a narrow space in the wrist called – you guessed it – the carpal tunnel. When the nerve is squashed, it gradually causes numbness and tingling in the fingers, particularly the thumb and first two fingers, since they are the ones supplied by this particular nerve. Reducing the dose of oestrogen usually helps and then everything goes back to normal.

WEIGHT GAIN

Although weight gain was a feature of the old high-dose pills used in the past, it is very unusual on the modern low-dose pills we use today. If it occurs, it may be for three reasons. Firstly, water retention can sometimes occur, due to oestrogen, in which case a lower-dose pill can be tried. Progestogens can cause an increase in appetite, which can obviously lead to an increase in weight. This is unusual on low-dose pills, and is even less likely with the new progestogens, so it may be worth changing to one of the newest pills as an experiment. The third and most likely reason is that you have simply been eating too much! I think there is a tendency among some women to feel 'now I'm on the pill, I'm bound to put on weight' and then to let themselves go and eat twice as much as usual. Or just to blame the pill when they have come back from holiday, or even worse, after Christmas!

HEADACHES/MIGRAINES

Simple headaches and migraines may both be aggravated by water retention, and therefore less oestrogen, or progestogen dominance, is usually the answer.

If they occur only, or to a much greater extent, in the pill-free week, you should simply not have one, i.e. just go straight from one packet to the next. This is likely to mean that you will not have a withdrawal bleed, but that doesn't matter. In some women, the drop in hormone levels during the pill-free week seems to bring on headaches or migraines. Tricycling is a good compromise, so that you take three or four packets in a row, and only have three or four pill-free weeks a year in which to have your headaches.

Headaches or migraines occurring in the last week of a triphasic pill will usually be dealt with by changing to a monophasic pill (one with the same dose throughout the packet).

If there is still a problem and you have tried all the above, the general rule is to try the lowest-dose pill possible, which does not give breakthrough bleeding.

Migraine: special cases

If your migraine is so bad that you have to regularly take specific medication for it containing a substance called ergotamine (as opposed to simple painkillers like aspirin or paracetamol), then you should not take the Combined Pill. This is because ergotamine constricts the blood vessels supplying the brain, which might make a thrombosis more likely. Migraine sufferers are already at a slightly increased risk of having a stroke, and this does not help matters. The pill might increase this risk slightly again, and although the chance of this happening on modern low-dose pills is extremely small, it would not be wise to tempt providence on a regular basis.

If you develop migraine for the first time ever while on the pill, or a migraine which is very severe and just gets worse and worse for a long time, you would be best advised to stop the pill, as this suggests that you are very sensitive to its effects.

If you have, or have ever had, what is called focal migraine, you should not take the Combined Pill at all. There is a great deal of confusion amongst both women and doctors as to what is and what is not focal migraine. Focal migraine is *not* the normal type, where you get a dreadful headache, often on one side of the head, nausea and/or vomiting, aversion to light, flashing lights in front of your eyes, blurring and therefore disrupted sight. For a migraine to be focal, you have to have a temporary paralysis, numbness or marked tingling in one side of your body, i.e. one arm and one leg on the same side, or just one arm or one leg. Focal migraine also includes a transient difficulty in speaking and a loss of vision specifically related to one side only, as though a piece of card had been placed over half the field of vision. The other visual aspect is so-called 'tunnel vision' where you feel as though you are looking through a small central hole, with everything around it dark, like looking through a tunnel, in fact. If you ever get any of these symptoms, you should stop the pill immediately and see your doctor. Unless some other explanation can be found, you should never take any oestrogen-containing medication again.

In all these circumstances, progestogen-only contraception can safely be used (see Chapters 5 and 6).

RAISED BLOOD PRESSURE

Some women do develop raised blood pressure due to the pill, which is why your blood pressure should be checked at least once a year while you are taking it. If your doctor is the type who just leaves your prescription with the receptionist and never sees you while you are on the pill, I suggest you find a new one.

You should bear in mind that blood pressure is not static, and changes all the time. It can be affected by stress, and so can go up and down depending on how you feel. This means that your blood pressure should be checked several times, not just once, and on different days, before it is stated that it really is high. And there are degrees of 'highness'. Blood pressure has two components, called the systolic and the diastolic. Systolic blood pressure reflects the pressure generated when the heart muscle contracts at each beat, while the diastolic measures the pressure when the heart is relaxed. Of the two, the diastolic is the more important, because obviously it is more serious if the pressure is high even when the heart is supposed to be relaxed.

Blood pressure is noted as two figures, written like a fraction, with the systolic first, or at the top, and the diastolic second, or at the bottom. So the classic textbook blood pressure would be written as 120/80. There is a wide range of blood pressure which is considered normal. Thus, the systolic can reach up to 140, and the diastolic can reach 90 before anyone is really worried. You can also have low readings, for example 90/60, which are considered normal. Low blood pressure is not dangerous, though you may find you feel faint when you stand up suddenly!

A blood pressure which is consistently around 140/90 would be a reason for changing to the lowest-dose pill possible, preferably containing one of the new progestogens as well. If it goes higher than that, you will need to consider coming off the Combined Pill and perhaps changing to a progestogen-only method.

DEPRESSION

Depression is always a difficult symptom to study. Most people feel 'depressed' occasionally, but some people are affected severely, such that it seriously disrupts their lives. So many things can make a person depressed that it is often difficult to know what was the real cause. After all, if you are on the pill and you lose your job, which was it that made you depressed? That is a simple example, but because people always look for an easy way to try and get rid of depression, women are bound to think of the pill.

Having said that, some women really do find that they feel 'happier' when they come off the pill, and may be helped by a change in type. The pills which contain the newer progestogens are likely to be the best from this point of view, since changing to a less 'progestogen-dominant' pill, or just one with a different progestogen, has sometimes been known to help. The new progestogens do not have 'progestogenic' side effects, so they should give the best results.

Another possibility is to try vitamin B6. A study has found that, of women who feel depressed on the pill, some have lower than normal blood levels of this vitamin. If such women (but not the ones with a normal blood level) are given vitamin B6, their depression improves. It is not usually possible to have your blood level of vitamin B6 measured, so it is simpler to just take vitamin B6 for a while and see what happens. A dose of 50 mg per day should be plenty. As always, you need to try this for at least two months before you can say whether or not it is helping.

Women on triphasic pills often find they get a sort of pre-menstrual syndrome in the last week of the packet, when they may also feel depressed. This will usually stop if you change to a monophasic pill (same dose all month).

LOSS OF LIBIDO

This means a loss of interest in sex, which, of course, makes taking the pill rather academic. Once again, it is always difficult to say whether it is the pill or something else which is causing it.

Top-of-the-list causes include stress, overwork, guilt, and 'falling out of love' with one's partner. Since just about everyone I meet nowadays says they are stressed and overworked, I wonder how many people can really blame their loss of sex drive on the pill.

Having said that, it is always worth a try. Once again, the best choice will be a pill containing one of the new progestogens, or even just a change to a more 'oestrogenic' pill.

If nothing seems to be helping, you may want to try coming off the pill and seeing what happens. Unfortunately, all too often, there is still no improvement, which is when you have to face the fact that there is some other cause. Think about the ones I mentioned above and see if one or more of them could apply to you. It might be helpful to see your doctor and perhaps be referred for psychosexual counselling.

DRYNESS DURING SEX

This really is related to loss of interest in sex, but may sometimes be separate, i.e. a woman can want to make love, but just finds she is dry. It may help to change to a pill containing one of the new protestogens, or a more 'oestrogenic' pill. However, if this does not help, bear in mind the discussion in the last section. Some women find that if the problem is temporary, for example they know they are going through a stressful time which will improve, it helps to use a lubricant, like KY jelly, which can be bought over the counter at the chemist.

INCREASE IN BODY HAIR

The medical term for excess hair is hirsutism. It can occur in women who are not on the pill and is more obvious, of course, in women who have dark hair. In rare cases this can be due to the pill, in which case it is a progestogen effect. It can be solved by changing to a more oestrogenic pill, or, better still, to a brand which contains one of the new progestogens as well as 30 micrograms of oestrogen. In fact, these newer pills are so good for this condition that women who develop it while not on the pill are often given one of these brands as treatment, whether or not they need contraception.

GREASY HAIR

This may be due to the progestogen, so an 'oestrogen-dominant' brand should help, or one of the brands containing the new progestogens. Even if you do choose one of those, you will find oestrogen helpful, so I would expect Marvelon or Minulet/Femodene to be better than Mercilon.

ACNE

If acne occurs on the pill, it is also a progestogenic effect. Changing to an 'oestrogen-dominant' pill or, even better, to a brand containing one of the new progestogens will help (preferably with 30 micrograms of oestrogen). Once again, these new pills have proved so successful that they are often used as treatment for women who suffer with bad acne.

CHLOASMA

This is a rare condition in which brown patches appear on the face. It also occurs in pregnancy. If this does happen to you, you will need to stop the pill (but please finish your packet and arrange an alternative method of contraception first, this is not life-threatening!). It is due to oestrogen, so changing brands, or even lowering the dose, will not make any difference. Sunbathing will make it much worse. It gradually fades, though it may never completely disappear. Unfortunately, if you become pregnant, it will get worse again, and similarly, if you develop it for the first time in pregnancy, you should not take the Combined Pill. You can still take the Progestogen-Only Pill.

PHOTOSENSITIVITY

A very small number of women find that being on the pill makes them intolerant of sunbathing. Instead of going their usual brown colour, they develop a red, blotchy rash. This can, of course happen even if you do not take the pill, but does seem to be slightly more common in pill users. The answer is to stop the Combined Pill, or to stop sunbathing altogether.

PROBLEMS WITH CONTACT LENSES

Even the slight water retention which may be caused by oestrogen can sometimes affect the shape of the eye and make contact lenses uncomfortable. Firstly, you should make sure you are taking the lowest-dose pill possible (i.e. that does not cause breakthrough bleeding). If you still have problems, you should see your contact lens specialist, as it may simply be a matter of altering the prescription slightly, or perhaps changing from hard lenses to soft lenses. Nowadays it is unusual for women to find it impossible to combine the pill and contact lenses, but it may require a little perseverance.

PREMENSTRUAL SYNDROME (PMS)

In theory, no woman should ever get PMS while on the pill, because the pill stops you ovulating, and therefore stops you menstruating (remember you are just having artificial withdrawal bleeds). The exception to this is triphasic pills, which mimic the so-called natural cycle so closely that they actually give women PMS who didn't have it before! So, if you are getting PMS-like symptoms (breast tenderness, bloating, depression) on a triphasic pill, try changing to a monophasic one (same dose all month) and you are very likely to improve.

Although the majority of women find their PMS is improved once they go on the pill (monophasic), some do not. It is worth trying a pill with one of the new progestogens, and also lowering the dose as much as possible. There is nevertheless a very small 'hard core' of women who will not be helped, or seem to actually be worse off on the pill. Depending on how much it disrupts your life, you may want to come off the pill, use a non-hormonal method of contraception and seek help for your PMS. There are many theories about what causes PMS, and even more proposed treatments. None of them work for everyone, but all of them help some women. Keep an open mind and be prepared to try several before finding one that helps you.

NAUSEA

This is quite common during the first couple of months of pill taking, but usually stops after that. If it does not, there are a couple of things to try. Nausea is usually related to oestrogen, so try a lower-dose pill. Some women find that nausea is not a problem if they take their pill at night. Conversely, you may find the opposite to be true. It is worth a change of timing to see if it helps. Taking any medication on an empty stomach can make people feel sick, so check whether this might not apply in your case.

A less common problem is nausea (or other side effects) which may be due to a colouring used in a pill. Allergies to colour additives do occur, the best known being tartrazine, which is a yellow colouring. It is sometimes worth changing brand, keeping the formulation the same and seeing if it helps. For example, Microgynon is yellow, while Ovranette, an identical pill, is white. Some women do find they are happier on a white rather than a coloured pill, even though the hormone content and type are the same.

VAGINAL DISCHARGE

Some women find that the amount of their 'normal' discharge is increased on the pill. This type of discharge is usually white or colourless, and does not cause itching or odour. If you notice an itchy or smelly discharge, it is most likely to be an infection of some kind, and you are best advised to have a check-up in a genitourinary medicine ('special') clinic.

The pill can give you an increase in non-infective discharge, by causing what is known as a cervical erosion or ectopy. This is a harmless condition of the cervix, which happens to be more common in women who are young, pregnant or taking the Combined Pill.

It simply means that the soft, columnar cells which line the inside of the womb have decided to spread outwards on to the surface of the cervix. These cells have a good blood supply, so they give a reddish appearance; this is why, when it was first noticed, it was described as looking like a graze, or 'erosion'. As well as a good blood supply, these cells have a large number of mucus-producing glands amongst them, and therefore they produce discharge.

The condition is harmless, but can be a nuisance. As mentioned earlier, it can occur in any young woman, regardless of whether she is on the pill, but the Combined Pill (not the Progestogen-Only Pill) does make it more likely.

If it is a nuisance, it can be treated quite easily by freezing the surface of the cervix (cryotherapy). This only takes a couple of minutes and is done in an outpatient clinic, so you don't go into hospital. However, if it is a big problem, you may wish to consider changing to a progestogen-only method, since if you stay on the Combined Pill it may recur.

THRUSH (CANDIDA, MONILIA)

This is a yeast infection which often causes itching and a creamy white discharge. It is extremely common, especially in hot, humid conditions, or when a woman is run down, for example during a cold or just prior to a period. It also occurs with monotonous regularity if a woman takes antibiotics.

The yeast is present in the vaginas of all women, only normally it is kept in check by the bacteria in the vagina, and by the woman's immune system. If her immune system is weakened (for example by having to deal with an infection elsewhere) or if she takes antibiotics (which kill off the bacteria), then thrush finds conditions to its liking and goes wild. Another way of helping thrush to multiply is to make the normally acidic vaginal environment (which it doesn't like) become more alkaline (which it likes). This can happen if you use bubble baths and perfumed soaps.

Thrush is normally quite simple to cure, the commonest treatment being a course of Canesten pessaries and cream. Now there is even a single pill you can take for thrush, called Diflucan, which is as effective as the pessaries and cream, but less messy. It is, however, no better at preventing recurrences.

Many women, and many doctors, are convinced that the pill makes thrush more likely, though this has not been shown to be the case in scientific studies. Thrush is very common, and pill taking is very common, so it is inevitable that there will be an overlap. The majority of women find that stopping the pill does not prevent them from getting thrush.

However, there are some women whose lives are plagued by thrush. They have it every month, it comes back as fast as it goes away. In these cases, I feel it is worth stopping the pill as an experiment (ANYTHING would be worth trying ...). At least that way the woman will feel better because she will know for certain whether it makes any difference, and it has to be said that occasionally coming off the pill does seem to help.

CRAMPS IN THE LEGS

This is a very common complaint among women on the pill, especially when they first start. It usually seems to wear off after a couple of months. If the pain is severe and the leg is swollen, you should see your doctor to make sure that you do not have a deep vein thrombosis (DVT), in which case you would need to stop the pill (see Chapter 3). However, this is very unlikely, and it is far more likely that there is no serious cause.

Varicose veins can cause pain in the legs, and if you are developing them, you should try not to stand still for long periods, nor wear high-heeled shoes. The pill does not cause varicose veins, contrary to popular mythology.

No one really knows why some women do get occasional cramps in the legs when they are on the pill, but they do not seem to have any sinister significance. Usually they just go away on their own, again for no apparent reason.

GALLSTONES

There is a link between the pill and gallstones, in that the pill seems to speed up their formation, if you were going to get them anyway. So it does not cause them, but it can make them become obvious more quickly. However, if you have had a cholecystectomy (removal of the gall bladder) due to gallstones, there is no reason why you cannot take the pill. After all, without a gall bladder, no more gallstones can form, so there is no longer any risk due to the pill.

THE IMMUNE SYSTEM

The effects of the pill on the immune system are poorly understood, not least because the immune system itself is still pretty much a mystery. Allergies and eczema seem to be more common in pill users, though one cannot be certain whether that might not be the case simply because women with allergies find other methods even worse. For example, spermicides, which are used in conjunction with sheaths and caps, are a common cause of allergy. Thus a woman who has a tendency to allergies or eczema might choose the pill because she has already found out that she reacts to spermicides, or is worried that she might.

Asthma does not appear to be affected by the pill, and

indeed the pill seems to improve some immune-related conditions, such as rheumatoid arthritis. Others, such as a condition known as systemic lupus erythematosus (SLE), are made worse. In general, if you suffer from a condition which affects the immune system, you should check with your specialist about the possible effects of the pill. The science of immunology changes too rapidly for anything very meaningful to be said in a book, especially of this type.

A WORD ABOUT TRIPHASIC PILLS

You may have noticed that throughout this chapter, triphasic pills have been mentioned again and again as a cause of problems and side effects. In my opinion, they really are more trouble than they are worth. They were introduced as a concept to try and reduce the level of progestogen in the pill as much as possible, while still maintaining good cycle control. However, they have since been entirely superseded by the new, monophasic pills containing the new progestogens, which do all that is needed without having to change the dose three times a month.

Triphasics are more complicated to take, because of the three different doses, and therefore have been shown to cause more pill-taking muddles, which can result in pregnancies. They are inconvenient, because if you want to skip a period, you have to know that you should keep taking the last row of the packet until you want to bleed. Many women do not realise this, and try to just run the two packets together, which is of no use, since the dose at the beginning is lower than that at the end. If you manage to do it correctly, you will use up your packets very fast, since the remaining portion is of no use to you. The alternative is to choose a monophasic pill which has the same composition as the last week of the packet, but this also is not always successful, and again means extra visits to your doctor.

Another annoying feature of triphasics is their tendency to cause premenstrual-syndrome-like symptoms. Breast tenderness, bloating, depression and headaches are all quite common in the last week of the packet. Women often have them but do not mention it to their doctor because they think it is normal. After all, they had this when they were not on the pill, and they forget that they are not having real periods, and therefore real cycles, while they are taking it. In fact, the pill, if it is the same dose all month, should *relieve* most women's PMS, which is a positive benefit. It seems silly to remove two of the benefits women can actually notice while on the pill – being able to skip periods at will, and getting rid of their PMS.

While I would not suggest that you stop your triphasic if you are perfectly happy on it, I do not recommend them as pills to start on, and if you are having any of the above-mentioned problems, a change to a monophasic pill will almost certainly give an improvement.

IN CONCLUSION

I hope this chapter has helped to sort out any annoying problems you may be experiencing on the pill, or are worried about. Inevitably, a book of this size cannot cover everything, but I have tried to include all the common problems, as well as the well-documented rarer ones. For more information, you may want to read *The Pill* by John Guillebaud (see Further Reading). Ultimately, however, you should seek advice from your doctor or family planning clinic.

4

TAKING THE PILL
– THE PRACTICALITIES

The Combined Pill (COC) is a very effective method of contraception, with a failure rate of only 0.5–1 per 100 women years. This means that if 100 women take the pill for a year, at most only one will become pregnant. However, like all methods, it needs to be used correctly.

It is unfortunate that women are bombarded with information about taking the pill, which can be downright contradictory. The manufacturers' leaflets give different instructions from the leaflets produced by the Family Planning Association (FPA) – and since the FPA leaflets have also been modified in the last couple of years, it is quite possible to see two FPA pill leaflets which say two different things, both of which will be different from the manufacturer's instructions. No wonder women are confused and mistakes occur.

There are several reasons for these differences. Basically they can be explained under the general principle of 'knowledge increases with time', hence each new set of pill rules is based on advances in our knowledge about how the pill works. The problems arise when the old rules are still around after the new ones have been announced.

Pharmaceutical companies are always the last to change their information sheets, but this is not entirely their fault. When a company applies for a licence to bring a pill on to the market, the information sheet they supply at that time becomes a legal document. If they want to change the information sheet, they have to virtually apply for a new licence. This is extremely time-consuming and costly, so it is not surprising that they often just don't bother. However, this does mean that the information which comes with each of your pill packets may be years out of date.

HOW TO TAKE THE PILL

Pills come in blister packs, usually containing 21 pills. They often have the days of the week printed against the pills, to help you remember whether you have taken one on a particular day. This does, of course, depend on you starting by choosing a pill which corresponds to the current day, i.e. if you start your pill on a Wednesday, but push out a pill which corresponds to Sunday, then you cannot blame anyone when you get confused a week later! Some manufacturers have really gone out of their way to try and be helpful, and even ask you to note which day you always start your packet (see the pictures below and overleaf)

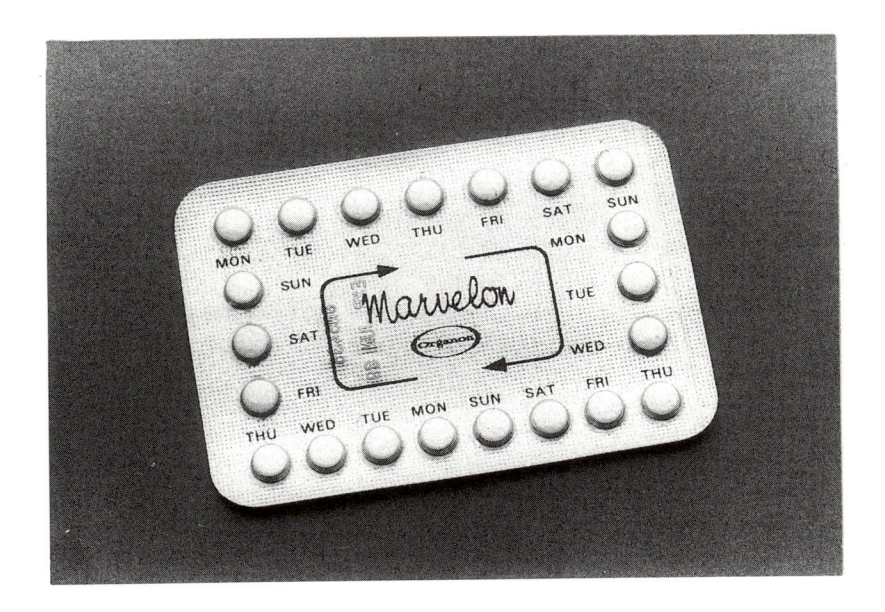

Figure 4.1

The least helpful packaging is the type where you have numbers instead of days printed on the back. This makes it much more difficult to tell whether you have forgotten to take one.

Basically, you take one pill a day until you have finished the packet. With the COC, the timing is not critical, as long as you do not let more than 36 hours go by from the time you took the last one, i.e. you can be up to 12 hours late taking your pill without any worries.

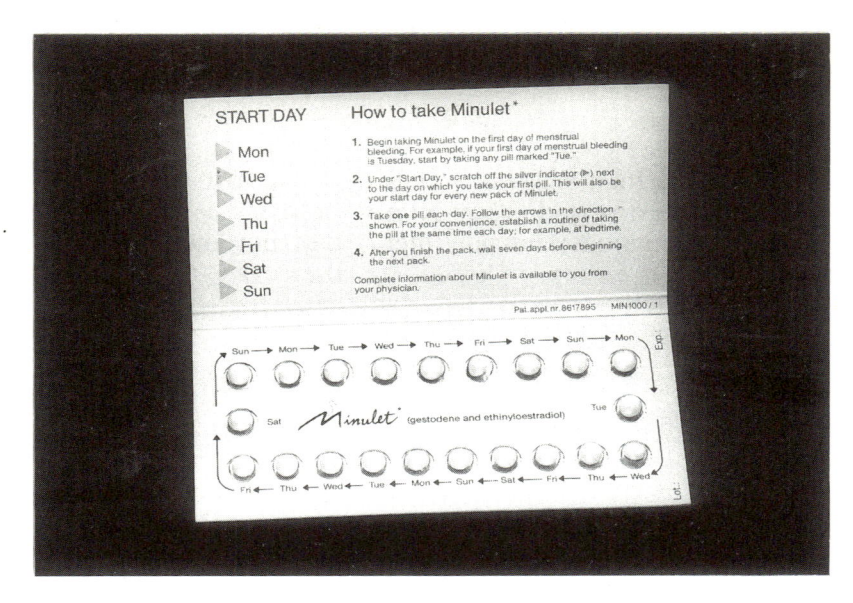

Figure 4.2 Minulet packets have clear instructions and days of the week printed against each pill.

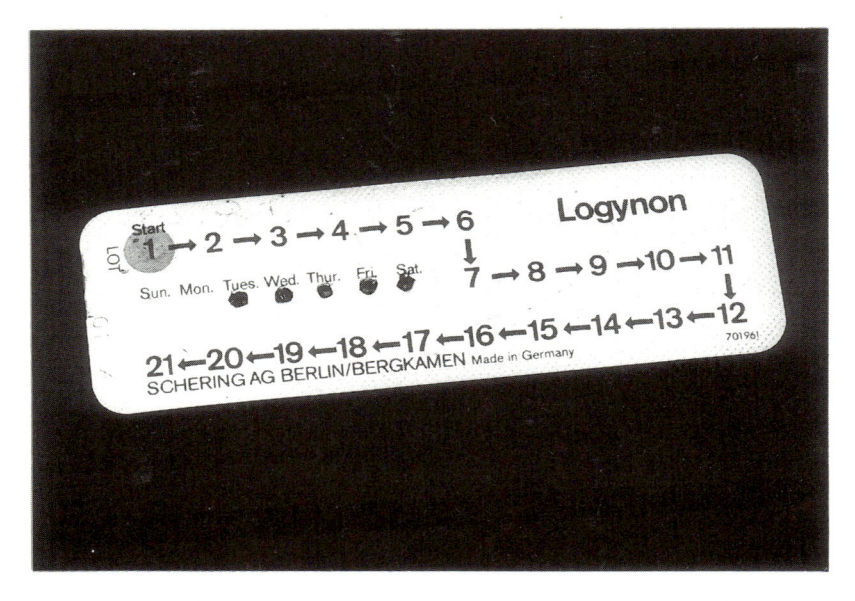

Figure 4.3 Numbers instead of days printed on a pill packet can make it more difficult to tell whether you have forgotten to take a pill.

62

When you have finished the packet, you have exactly seven days' break, and you start your next packet on the eighth day. Most women have their withdrawal bleed ('period') during the gap; some women never have withdrawal bleeds, others miss them occasionally. It doesn't matter. Withdrawal bleeds are nothing more than artificial bleeds designed to make you feel you have had a period. They do not, however, have the same meaning as periods; missing them does not mean you are pregnant, and conversely, you can easily have a withdrawal bleed while you are actually pregnant. The important thing to realise here is: if you do not see a withdrawal bleed, make sure you restart your pills on the eighth day as usual, consult your doctor if you are worried, but meanwhile, keep taking the tablets! Otherwise, you may really become pregnant when you weren't before.

There is one pill (Minylin) which contains 22 tablets in a packet and then you only have a six day break. In addition, there are a few ED (Every Day) preparations, which contain 28 tablets. These packets include seven 'dummy' pills, which do not contain any hormones. The advantage is that you don't have to remember to restart the next packet after the seven-day break, because you take a pill every day.

HOW TO START TAKING THE PILL

In general, you should start the pill on the first day of your period, and you will then be protected straight away. No additional contraceptive precautions will be necessary. (By additional precautions, I mean the sheath, diaphragm/cap or abstinence.) In fact this is still true if you start the pill on the second or third day of your period.

This is a relatively recent change in the rules, and is due to the realisation that we have been much too cautious in the past. There does not appear to be any chance of a pregnancy being able to occur if you start right at the beginning of a period.

However, if you start after the third day, you will need to use additional contraceptive precautions for the next seven days.

Logynon ED is different, because you are advised to start your packet with the 'dummy' pills. This means that you will need to use additional precautions for seven days, even though you start on the first day of your period.

Trinovum ED is more sensible, because the dummy pills are put last, and you do, in fact, start on active pills. This means that you are protected straight away, as with ordinary pills.

If you have had a miscarriage or abortion, you should start the pill on the same or next day. No additional precautions will be necessary.

After having a baby, it is advisable to wait until the third week after delivery, because there is an increased risk of thrombosis (blood clots) during pregnancy and for a short time afterwards. It is obviously best not to add on the slight risk due to the pill. However, ovulation has not been known to occur before the end of the fourth week after delivery, so if you start on or around the twenty-first day, you will be protected without requiring additional precautions. Of course, all this only applies if you are not breastfeeding: if you are, you should not be using the Combined Pill, but can safely use the Progestogen-Only Pill (see Chapters 5 and 7).

If you are changing from one Combined Pill to another, provided they are of equivalent dosage, you just start it after your normal seven-day break, without the need for additional precautions. (For these purposes, you need only compare the oestrogen dose, and 30 and 35 micrograms can be considered

Figure 4.4 Starting routines for the Combined Pill.

	When to start	Extra precautions
Starting pill for first time or after a break	1st, 2nd or 3rd day of period	No
	After 4th day	Yes, for 7 days
Changing to COC of same or higher dose	After normal 7-day break	No
Changing to lower-dose COC	Straight after last pill of previous packet, i.e. no 7-day break	No
	If normal 7-day break	Yes, for 7 days
From POP to COC	1st day of period (no break)	No
From POP to COC when woman has no periods on POP	Any time (no break)	No
After an abortion or miscarriage	Same or next day	No
After childbirth (if not breastfeeding)	Between 21st and 28th day after delivery	No

N.B. Rules for Logynon ED are different, please see text.

to be equivalent.) The same applies if you are changing from a lower to a higher-dose pill.

However, if you are changing from a higher- to a lower-dose pill, you should skip the pill-free week and just go straight on to your new pill, i.e. if you stop your current pill on Wednesday, start taking the new one the next day (in this case Thursday). If you do this, you will not need to use any additional precautions. However, if for some reason a straight switch is inconvenient or impossible, you can still have a seven-day break, but you will then need to use additional precautions for a week.

If you are changing from the Progestogen-Only Pill (POP), you should change on the first day of a period, without any additional precautions. Women who do not have periods (and are therefore not ovulating) while on the POP can just do a straight switch at any time, without needing to use extra precautions.

WHAT TO DO WHEN YOU FORGET A PILL

This is another area in which new research findings have led to a change in the rules. In order to understand this, you need to know a little more about the pill-free week.

Many women are puzzled by the fact that they are still protected during their pill-free week, even though they are not taking any pills. Although it is true that you *are* protected, their concern is actually not far off the mark. Figure 4.5 shows what happens to the levels of natural hormones, produced by the ovary during the pill-free week. As you can see, the level rises quite rapidly, but drops again when you restart pill taking on the eighth day. However, if you were to forget to restart, the hormone levels would continue to rise, and might well reach a level which would trigger the LH surge (see Chapter 1) and cause ovulation. Even being late by a couple of days might be enough to allow pregnancy. The same, of course, applied to forgetting pills at the end of a packet. If you don't take, say, the last three pills, and then you add on your normal pill-free week, you will effectively have had a gap of 10 days during which your hormone levels could be getting seriously out of control.

Most women don't realise that it is so very important not to miss pills at the beginning or end of a packet. They are usually much more concerned about the pill they missed in the middle. What do you think is likely to happen if you miss your twelfth pill, for example? Your ovaries are completely dormant after seven days of pill taking, and they are likely to need at least seven days 'off' before pregnancy could occur. So the result of missing your twelfth pill is: nothing, except a lot of unnecessary anxiety. Of course, if you start forgetting several pills at a time, you are more likely to be at risk, but there is still nothing as dangerous as prolonging the pill-free week.

This knowledge has led to a change in the rules for missed pills. The new recommendations are as follows:

If you are less than 12 hours late taking a pill, just take the one you forgot and carry on as normal. Take your next pill at the usual time, even if this means you are taking two pills in one day. No other precautions are necessary.

If you are more than 12 hours late, take the one you forgot straight away, and then the next one at your usual time. You should now assume you are not fully protected for the next seven days, so you will need to use additional precautions. *Also*, if you have fewer than seven pills left in your packet, you should skip the pill-free interval, and just go straight on to the next packet the day after you finish the current one. Obviously, if you have already weakened the effect of the pill, the last thing you need is to stop it completely for seven days. This means you may not have a withdrawal bleed that month, but, as I have already explained, that does not matter. If you are taking a

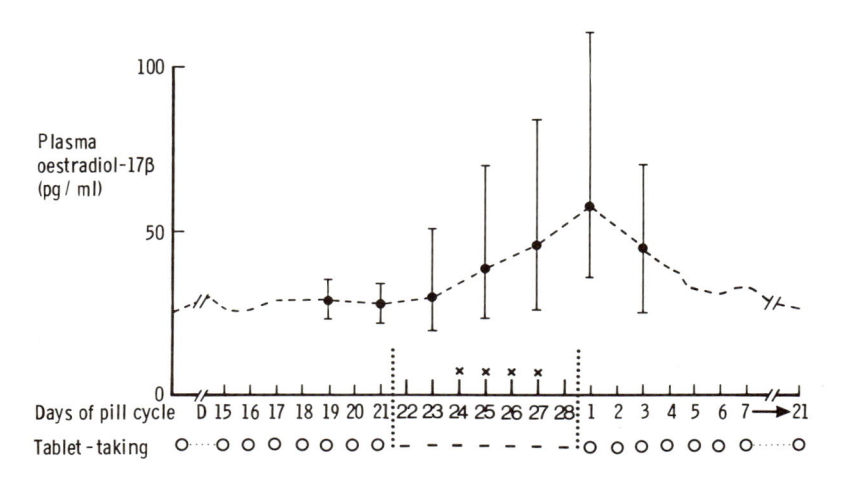

Figure 4.5 Levels of plasma oestradiol; before, during and after the pill free week.

(Source: *Contraception: Science and Practice* Marcus Filshie and John Guillebaud *see* Further Reading)

triphasic pill, the chances are that you will have some breakthrough bleeding, because the dose at the beginning of the packet is lower than at the end. Once again, although a nuisance, this does not matter.

If you are taking an Every Day (ED) pill, you need to check to see whether you have more than seven active pills left in your packet. If you do not, you should make sure that you do not take the dummy pills this cycle, and just start a new packet (taking active pills, of course).

If you realise that you have forgotten to restart your packet after the pill-free week, and have had sex in the last couple of days without using additional precautions, you should consider asking for the 'morning after pill' (see Chapter 7).

IF YOU HAVE A STOMACH UPSET

Essentially, the rules are the same as for missed pills, which is effectively what is happening. You should consider a pill to have been 'missed' if you vomited within four hours of taking it. You should try to take another one, but if you are vomiting frequently there may not be much point. If you have severe diarrhoea, it is more difficult to tell just when the pill may have disappeared, and whether it is likely to have been properly absorbed. It is probably best to play safe and assume you have missed pills on any days that it occurs.

You should use extra precautions for the duration of the stomach upset, and for seven days afterwards. Once again, if you have fewer than seven active pills left, you should skip the pill-free week.

IF YOU HAVE TO TAKE OTHER MEDICINES

There are two main ways in which other medications can interfere with the pill, and they have different implications. The first type of interference is through what is called **enzyme induction**. This means that the drug speeds up the action of the liver enzymes which destroy the hormones in the pill. As you might imagine, this means less pill left for you.

Fortunately not many women are likely to find themselves taking such medication. An important group, however, are those who suffer from epilepsy. All the drugs used to treat epilepsy interfere with the pill in this way, except one. The exception is sodium valproate (Epilim), and if you only need to take this, the advice here does not apply to you.

Another important group, though less common in this country, are those women who are being treated for tuberculosis with a drug called Rifampicin.

A list of enzyme-inducing drugs which interfere with the pill is given below. If you are in any doubt, check with your doctor. Sometimes your doctor may not be sure either, in which case he or she can ring a hospital pharmacy, or another useful source of information is likely to be the pill manufacturers themselves. A list of their names, addresses and telephone numbers is given at the end of this book.

If you are on long-term medication using an enzyme-inducing drug (and in the majority of cases this is likely to be so) you will probably need to take a higher-than-average dose of the pill. Traditionally, this has been done using 50-microgram pills. However, none of these contain the new progestogens, so you might wish to consider the idea of taking two lower-dose pills each day. For example, you could take two pills a day of Mercilon. This would give a total of 40 micrograms of oestrogen, plus 300 micrograms of desogestrel. You will know whether this dose is sufficient by watching out for any breakthrough bleeding. If you have none, you are OK. If you do have breakthrough bleeding, then you need more hormones, so you could take one Marvelon plus one Mercilon per day. This would give you 50 micrograms of oestrogen and 300 micrograms of desogestrel. If you still get breakthrough bleeding, you could take two Marvelons or two Minulets/Femodenes per day. This would increase the dose to 60 micrograms of oestrogen, with either 300 micrograms of desogestrel or 150 micrograms of gestodene. You just keep increasing the dose until you stop having breakthrough bleeding.

You do not need to worry about the high dose of hormones you are taking: since your liver is destroying them almost as fast as you can swallow them, you are not actually *using* that amount of hormone. All you are doing is allowing for the extra wastage: the dose your body actually makes use of will be the same as though you were on a normal-strength pill, if you were not taking the interacting medication.

In fact, under these circumstances, it is also recommended that you shorten your pill-free gap to four days, or even take three packets in a row before having a pill-free four-day gap. This is because you would be particularly vulnerable to the possibility of ovulation during the pill-free week, since the effect of the hormones does not last for so long.

Figure 4.6 Enzyme-inducing drugs.

Drugs used in the treatment of epilepsy
Barbiturates
Phenytoin
Primidone
Carbamazepine
Ethosuximide
(but *not* sodium valproate)

Antibiotics
Rifampicin

Antifungal drugs
Griseofulvin

Diuretics
Spironolactone

Strong sedatives/tranquillisers
Chloral hydrate
Dichloralphenazone
Chlorpromazine

N.B. You may need to check the packet to find the 'proper' name of the drug, as there are several trade names for each of these

An important point to remember is that if you stop taking an enzyme-inducing medicine, you still need the higher-dose pill for at least four weeks afterwards. This is because the effect takes a while to wear off.

If you take an enzyme-inducing medicine for only a short time, it may not be worth changing to a higher-dose pill. In that case, you should use extra precautions while you are taking the medication and for seven days afterwards, skipping the pill-free week if necessary.

The second type of interaction occurs with broad spectrum antibiotics, such as penicillin, the tetracyclines and neomycin. This interaction works in quite a different way, by killing off the bacteria which normally live in the gut. These bacteria are very useful in the enterohepatic cycle. This is simply the name used to describe the wanderings of oestrogen and progestogen from the gut to the liver and back again. What happens is this: oestrogen and progestogen are absorbed from the gut and travel to the liver. The liver enzymes attack them and convert a proportion into byproducts, which are then thrown back into the bowel as waste, waiting to be disposed of. However, the bacteria which live in the bowel can reconvert oestrogen into a useful form and it can then be reabsorbed into the blood and used. Unfortunately, they can do nothing for the progestogen, which just has to quietly await its fate.

This does mean that the bacteria are actually contributing to the amount of oestrogen which is available for the body to use. If these bacteria are wiped out by antibiotics, that oestrogen will disappear along with the progestogen, thus lowering the amount available to the body.

This effect is very small, but may be important in some women whose oestrogen levels are only just being maintained at an adequate level by the action of the bacteria. Such women may be at risk of pregnancy if they take these antibiotics. If only we knew in advance who they were.... Because it is not

THE ENTERO — HEPATIC CIRCULATION

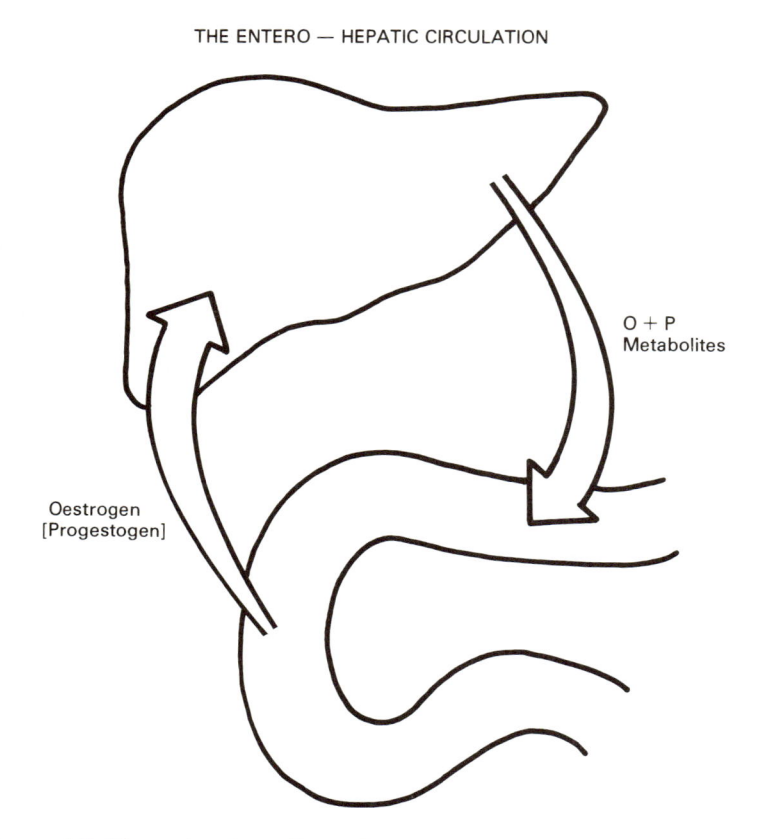

Figure 4.7 The enterohepatic cycle.

(Source: *Contraception: your questions answered* John Guillebaud *see* Further Reading)

possible to tell, all women are advised to use extra precautions while taking courses of these antibiotics, and for seven days afterwards, omitting the pill-free interval as described *ad nauseam* above. (I'm afraid these rules do become very repetitive.)

The good news is that if you take such antibiotics for a long time (for example tetracyclines for acne), you need only use extra precautions for the first four weeks. The plucky little bacteria become resistant to the antibiotics after about three or four weeks, and then it doesn't matter any more. In fact, if you have been on tetracycline for your acne for months, and then are started on the pill, you don't need to use extra precautions at all: the bacteria have already been resistant for ages. The important time to use extra precautions is if you are on the pill and then start a course of, for example, tetracycline, which you intend to use for several months. These are the circumstances under which you need to use extra precautions for the first month.

MOVING PERIODS

One of the advantages of being on the pill is that you can move your periods to suit you. If you are taking a monophasic pill, all you need to do is to skip the pill-free week. This means you will not have a period that month. Alternatively, if you only want to postpone your withdrawal bleed for a few days, or a week, just take extra pills until it becomes convenient to have a bleed, and then stop. No more weekends away carrying packets of tampons, no more holidays marred by a suitcase half full of sanitary towels.

If you are taking a triphasic pill, postponing withdrawal bleeds is not so easy (which is one of the reasons why I do not like them). In this case, what you have to do is to keep taking the last row of pills for as long as necessary. This may involve using up a lot of pill packets, since, of course, the remaining part is of little use to you. Apart from the wastage, it means you will run out of packets and have to go back for more sooner than usual – in itself a nuisance. If you try to just run the packets together, you will still bleed because the dose at the end is higher than the dose at the beginning.

It is perfectly safe to move your withdrawal bleeds around. After all, they are only artificial bleeds produced by stopping the pill. They mean nothing. You can even be pregnant and still have them. Nor is it necessary to bleed every month. There are no 'evil spirits' to be washed away. Nevertheless, some women do find that if they don't have their seven-day break, they feel bloated and uncomfortable. I am sure that some of this is psychological, but equally, the pill can cause slight water retention, and it may be that in some women it is enough to make them uncomfortable if they do not have a break (during which it presumably improves again). The majority of women do not have any problems skipping withdrawal bleeds occasionally.

WHY HAVE WITHDRAWAL BLEEDS AT ALL?

A very good question. Well, as I mentioned in the last section, many women do feel happier to see a bleed each month, and some do find that they feel bloated if they do not have a break from the pill. Indeed, the reason pill-free weeks are advised is actually because the man who invented the pill felt that women would be happiest seeing a regular, though artificial period. There was no scientific reason.

Having said that, it is of course now true that all the research studies looking at the pill have been done on women who had a pill-free week. We cannot be sure whether the findings would be exactly the same if the pill was taken continuously. Taking the pill without any breaks at all would mean taking three extra packets each year. Would this make any difference to long-term health risks? Nobody knows.

A few studies done using old, high-dose pills showed that the lowering of HDL cholesterol (see Chapter 1) caused by the pills was to some extent reversed during the pill-free week, and it was therefore suggested that the break might be useful in reducing the risks of cardiovascular disease. The newest pills do not have this effect on HDL cholesterol, nor any other significant metabolic effects. It seems less likely, therefore that the breaks are beneficial from this point of view.

On the opposing side are the disadvantages of the pill-free week. They lead to pill omissions (women forget to restart), and therefore to pregnancies. They result in withdrawal bleeds, which can be a nuisance. Some women get side effects, such as headaches or a kind of pre-menstrual syndrome, during them.

Continuous pill taking is actually recommended in some gynaecological conditions, such as endometriosis, where bleeding is to be discouraged. It is also often recommended for epileptic women, since hormone fluctuations may encourage fits to occur.

The disadvantages need to be balanced against the advantages, both real and theoretical. In the end, each woman must decide for herself, and this will partly depend on how many of the disadvantages of the pill-free week she has experienced.

As a compromise, the concept of tricycling has been developed.

TRICYCLING

This means taking three, or sometimes four packets without a break, and then stopping for a week. It is particularly recommended for women who get side effects related to the pill-free week, such as headaches which occur only or mostly at that time. It can also be useful for women who have heavy and/or painful withdrawal bleeds. In addition, it is recommended for women who are taking enzyme-inducing drugs, which reduce the effectiveness of the pill. By tricyling, the women only have to have the unpleasant effects of the pill-free week three or four times a year, instead of every month. And they still have the potential advantage of having some pill-free weeks rather than none at all. Once again, you do not have to have a specific side effect before you can tricycle – any woman can do this, if she chooses to.

BREAKS FROM THE PILL

Breaks from the pill are entirely unnecessary. There is no medical reason why you should need to stop to 'give your body a rest', whereas, in fact, if you think about it, every time you have a pill-free week, you are effectively having a break for seven days. The most depressing feature of breaks from the pill is that unwanted pregnancies occur – and that surely cannot be good for your health, either physically or psychologically.

MONITORING YOUR HEALTH WHILE YOU ARE ON THE PILL

Before you start the pill or, indeed, any method of contraception, your doctor should take details of your own medical and family history, to make sure there are no reasons why you should not use it, or have any investigations done before taking it. You should have your blood pressure checked and you should be weighed. You should have an opportunity to ask any questions, not just about the pill, but about any methods of contraception.

You should be seen three months after starting a new pill, so that any problems can be dealt with, any new questions asked, and your blood pressure checked again. Women often feel that 'minor' side effects are too trivial to ask a busy doctor about, which is why a three-month visit should automatically be made, so that you do not feel you are having to ask especially to be seen.

Once you are established and happy on a particular brand, you should be seen every six months. It is not good enough for a prescription just to be left for you to pick up. This gives you no opportunity to voice any worries or discuss any new side effects. Your blood pressure and weight should be checked at least once a year.

Women are often worried that they will have to be examined before they can go on the pill. That is certainly not true. However, you should have a cervical smear taken at least every three years, and an internal examination at the same time.

These are general principles, which apply not just to the Combined Pill, but to any method of hormonal contraception. If you are not receiving a satisfactory service from your doctor, or you cannot see a female doctor at your practice, you are entitled to see another doctor or family planning clinic for family planning services, even if you remain registered with your original GP.

The last few chapters have concentrated on the Combined Pill. However, not everyone can or wants to take oestrogen. Let us now look at other hormonal methods of contraception.

5

THE PROGESTOGEN-ONLY PILL

As its name implies, this type of pill contains no oestrogen, and therefore differs fundamentally from the Combined Pill. Unfortunately, it is often referred to as the 'mini-pill', which gives the impression that it may be a low-dose Combined Pill, which it is not. Throughout this book, I shall refer to the Progestogen-Only Pill as the POP.

The POP is, at present, greatly underused. This is mainly because not many women, or their doctors, actually know it exists. However, it is a very useful method of contraception, particularly for those women who either cannot or do not want to take oestrogen.

HOW DOES THE POP WORK?

The main difference between this pill and the Combined Pill (COC) is that it cannot be relied upon to stop ovulation (release of the egg). Studies have shown that 40 per cent of women who take this type of pill will continue to ovulate normally. Another 40 per cent will experience a disruption of ovulation, and the remaining 20 per cent do not ovulate at all.

You may be thinking that the POP presumably only works in the women who do not ovulate, but this is not true: it has other tricks up its sleeve.

The first of these is an effect on cervical mucus, making it thicker and more difficult for sperm to get through. Figure 5.1 on page 77 shows you greatly magnified photographs of cervical mucus. As you can see, normal mucus at mid-cycle, when you are most fertile, has very large gaps between the strands, allowing plenty of room for sperm to swim through. However, four hours after you have swallowed a POP, the strands form a dense mesh. The sperm are beating their heads against a brick wall. Now look at the third photograph; you will see it looks remarkably like the first one, of friendly mid-cycle mucus. Unfortunately, this is what happens if you are only 12 hours late taking the next pill. For this reason, the pill-taking regimen for the POP has to be much stricter than that for the COC, and you have to take it within three hours of the same time each day.

The other way in which the POP works is by reducing the size and number of the blood vessels in the lining of the womb, making it thin and less likely to allow implantation (the embedding of a fertilised egg) to take place. This acts as a 'fail safe' mechanism: even if a woman has ovulated, and a sperm has managed to battle its way through the cervical mucus, hopefully the effect on the lining will stop the pregnancy just in time.

HOW EFFECTIVE IS THE POP?

Because it does not guarantee to stop ovulation, the POP is not as effective as the Combined Pill. However, it does not compare badly, with a failure rate which ranges from 0.5 to 4 per cent. It improves with age, as does any method of contraception which allows you to ovulate – you ovulate less frequently as you get older, so the 'top-up' needed becomes less.

It is important to know the approximate failure rates which can be expected at different ages, because this may influence your decision as to whether to try it now, or wait till you are older. Figure 5.2 on page 78 shows a graph of failure rates with age. As you can see, over the age of 30, the failure rate is quite acceptable, at under 2 per cent (this means that if 100 women use the POP for a year, two will become pregnant). However, under the age of 25, where the failure rate is 4 per cent, the graph rises rapidly. Although not many young women have used the POP, so accurate figures are not available, it is thought the failure rate is much higher, probably around 10 per cent (i.e. 10 out of 100 women would become pregnant in a year).

So the POP is best suited to women over the age of 25, and preferably over the age of 30. In this discussion 35 is an

(b)

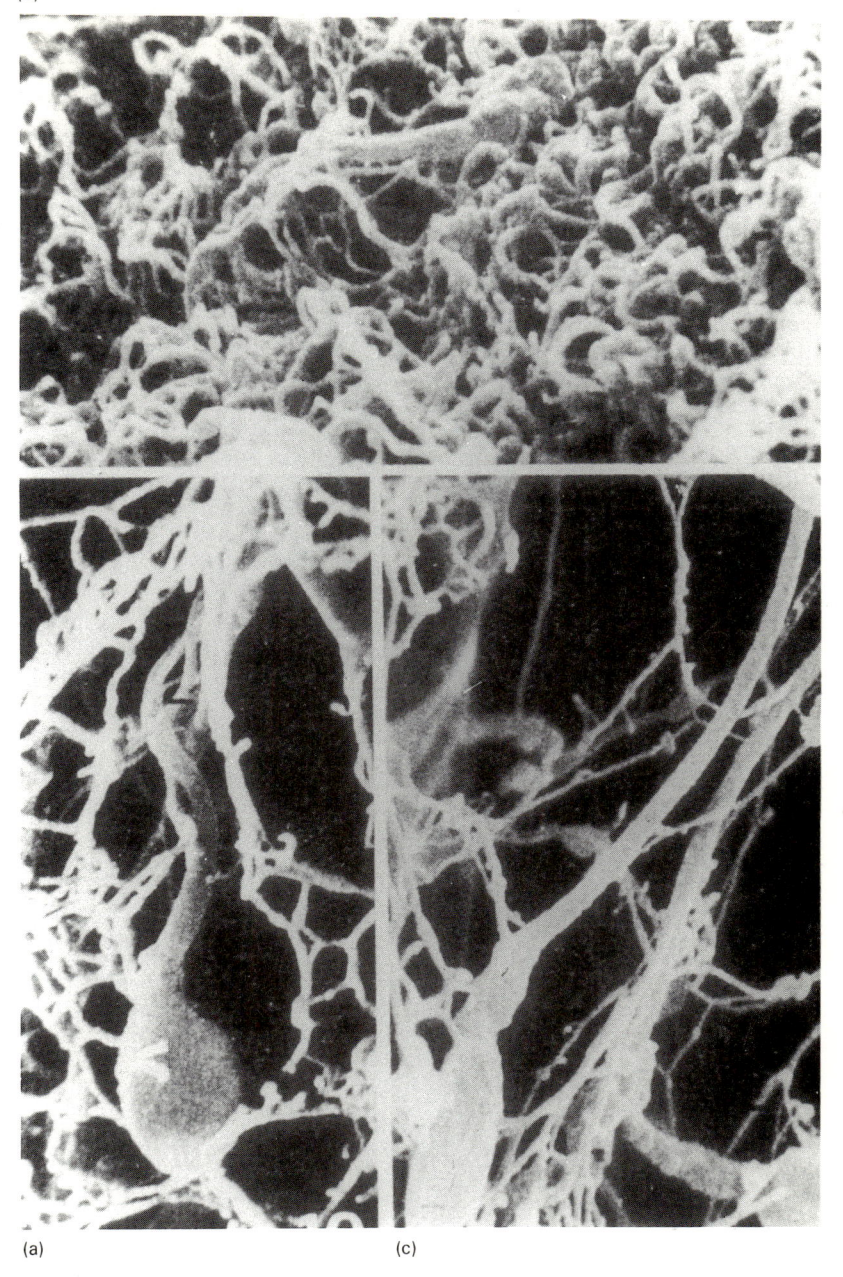

(a) (c)

Figure 5.1 Cervical mucus (greatly magnified) (a) is normal mid-cycle mucus (b) is mucus four hours after POP has been taken, and (c) is mucus 36 hours after last POP.

FAILURE RATES FOR PROGESTOGEN ONLY PILLS
BY AGE OF USER

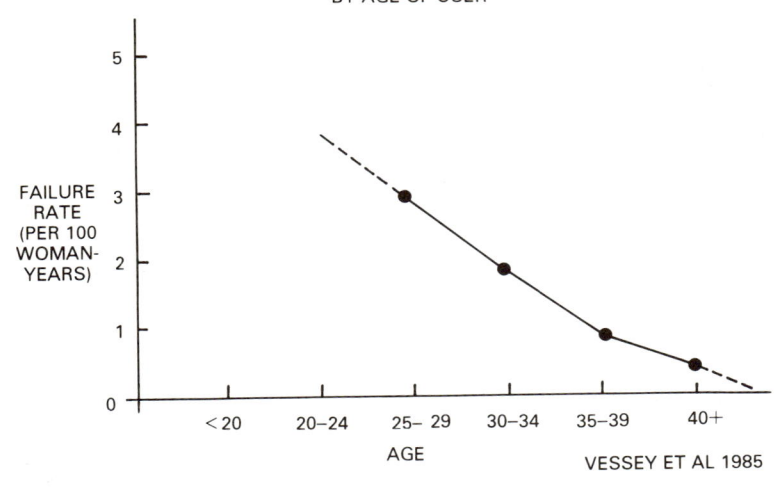

Figure 5.2 Graph shows failure rates for Progestogen-Only Pills by age of user.

important age; at this age, the failure rate is comparable to that of the COC (1 per cent), so it is ideal for women who smoke and therefore have to give up the COC by then (see below).

WHAT TYPES OF PROGESTOGEN-ONLY PILLS ARE AVAILABLE?

Figure 5.3 shows you the main brands in use, and the table below shows their composition. As you can see, the dose of progestogen used in each of these brands is lower than that used in Combined Pills.

Composition of Progestogen-Only Pills.

Femulen	Ethynodiol diacetate	500 µg
Micronor/Noriday	Norethisterone	350 µg
Microval/Norgeston	Levonorgestrel	30 µg
Neogest	Norgestrel	75 µg

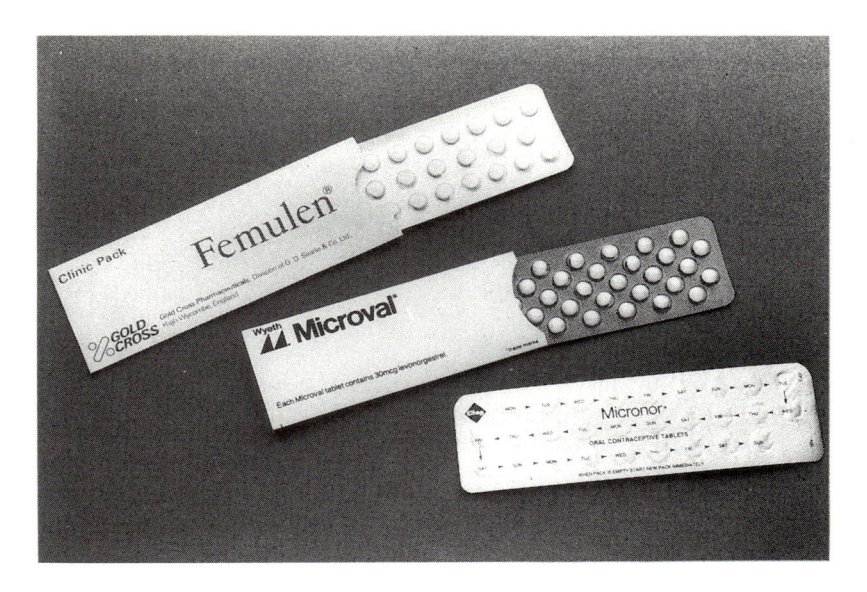

Figure 5.3 The main brands of Progestogen-Only Pills.

ADVANTAGES OF THE POP

The most important feature of the POP is that it contains no oestrogen. This means that if you have been advised not to take the Combined Pill because of your family history, your own medical history, or because you experienced side effects on it, you can almost certainly take the POP.

The POP does not affect blood pressure or increase the risk of heart disease. It does not affect blood clotting or the blood levels of HDL cholesterol, so a woman could still take it even if she had had a thrombosis (blood clot). This also means that there is no age limit for taking this pill, even if you smoke. Although smokers have to stop the Combined Pill at the age of 35, they can continue with the POP until the menopause. And even if you have to take tablets to lower your blood pressure, it is all right to take the POP.

The POP does not affect blood sugar, so it can safely be used by diabetics. Nor does it matter if you are very overweight; the POP will not make you put on any more, or increase the risk to your health.

In general, the side effects of the Combined Pill do not occur on the POP. So, if you had raised blood pressure on the

Combined Pill, you can still take the POP. If you suffer from headaches or migraine (including 'focal' migraine, see Chapter 3) or which became worse on the Combined Pill, you can take the POP. If you felt bloated, put on weight or had breast tenderness, you should find you improve on the POP. Women who develop chloasma (brown patches on the face) can take the POP. Although depression and loss of interest in sex are not usually oestrogenic side effects, if no brand of Combined Pill has improved matters, it is worth trying the POP; the dose of progestogen is so small, you may find that the effect disappears.

The POP can be safely used during breastfeeding. It does not stop the production of milk, nor does it have any effect on the baby. Because it is such a small dose, and only a tiny amount of that actually passes into the milk, it has been calculated that if a woman took the POP every day while breastfeeding for two years, at the end of that time the baby would have absorbed the equivalent of just one tablet. Breastfeeding itself has a slight contraceptive effect, so when a woman who is breastfeeding takes the POP, her protection against pregnancy becomes close to 100 per cent, i.e. better than that given by the POP alone.

There is no delay in the return of your fertility after stopping the POP, nor is there any need to stop taking it a few months before trying for pregnancy. Even if you fall into the small group of women who do not have periods on this type of pill (see below), they will return rapidly once you stop.

The POP has not been shown to have any effect, either good or bad, on any kind of cancer. Having said that, it must be added that not as many women have taken it and therefore it has not been as extensively researched as the Combined Pill. Nevertheless, what evidence there is is all in its favour (one study has even shown it to be perhaps slightly protective against breast cancer which, though unlikely to be very significant, is reassuring).

DISADVANTAGES OF THE POP

The pill-taking routine

One of its main disadvantages is that you have to take it at the same time (or at least within three hours of the same time) every day. So it is not for the absent-minded! With a little thought, however, most women can manage this if they want to. The time at which you take it is up to you, though you may hear that it is best to take it at about 6 p.m. This is based on the assumption that the majority of people make love at about 11 p.m., and that the blood levels of most tablets are at their highest a few hours after you have swallowed them. Now, firstly, the assumption about the time of lovemaking may not apply to you, and secondly, whatever the optimal time may be, the POP does work throughout 24 hours. Personally, I cannot think of a worse time to try and remember to do something regularly than 6 p.m. Where will you be: in the office, in the pub, on the bus, on the train? Certainly not in the same place every day, and almost certainly not in a place where it is easy to take your pill. It is better to aim lower and succeed than to try for the impossible and fail.

Taking pills at breakfast time suits many people, provided you do not get up very much later at weekends. An alternative may be to keep a set of pills in the office and take one when you arrive: this is likely to make weekend timekeeping easier. It is certainly a good idea to keep a spare packet at work or in your handbag, just in case you do forget. Some women have a digital watch and set the alarm to remind themselves to take their pills!

If you are a frequent traveller, time zone changes can be a problem. The solution is to make sure you take two pills within 24 hours, rather than risk taking a pill late. Remember, it is such a low dose that doubling it for a day is not going to do you any harm. And it is a good idea to keep a packet of pills permanently in your suitcase, so that you are not caught out if you forget to pack your current one.

One last point about the timing of the pill: when you decide on your regular time, try to avoid taking it actually around the time you would most often make love. After all, it will take a couple of hours to be fully absorbed, so you will, to some extent, be relying on yesterday's pill. There is only a small risk that it would not be as effective, but it seems sensible not to take that risk on a regular basis.

Period problems

As I have mentioned before, nearly half of the women who take the POP will have regular periods. However, about a fifth stop having periods altogether, and, naturally enough, become worried about pregnancy. In actual fact, such women are at least risk of becoming pregnant, because they are the small group who stop ovulating. This means you would be as well protected as if you were taking the Combined Pill, without the possible health risks or side effects. And it does not mean that you would have any extra difficulty becoming pregnant after stopping. However, of course, when it first happens there is the worry that you may have forgotten a pill, or had a stomach upset, and in fact become pregnant. Because of this possibility, you should have a pregnancy test about a week after your missed period. It if is negative, and your period still has not come, have another one a couple of weeks later. If it is still negative, then the most likely reason is that you have stopped ovulating, and you can relax. After that, of course, you know that you are very unlikely to become pregnant, so you do not need to keep having pregnancy tests.

It has to be said that not all women adjust well to the idea of not having periods, especially if they know that they are not always good at remembering to take their pill. Sometimes a change of brand is enough to bring the periods back, so you should discuss this with your doctor.

The main type of period problem caused by the POP (which happens to about 40 per cent of the women on it at some time) is irregular periods. This can range from infrequent periods, to periods every three weeks, to constant spotting. It can be very tiresome indeed, and unfortunately there is no way of predicting what is likely to happen in any individual case. Often this is what happens when a woman first starts taking the POP, and will settle down after a couple of months, so it is worth persevering. If there is still no improvement, a change of brand will sometimes help. There is very little science in this – whatever brand you are on, just changing to one of the others may improve matters.

In fact, the three types of period pattern I have described may happen to the same woman at different times. For example, she may have irregular periods for the first few months, after which they settle down for a year or several years. Then, for no apparent reason, she will either have irregular periods again, or may stop having them altogether for a while. Then they may become regular again and so on. No one really understands the reason for this, but the irregular periods seem to occur when the ovaries are slightly disrupted from their usual hormone-producing routine. When they settle down again, the woman has regular periods, and of course, if they stop ovulating, she stops having periods. (These things can also happen to a woman who is not using any type of hormonal contraception – I am sure many of you have experienced irregular periods occasionally when you are under stress or if you travel.)

Ovarian cysts

It does seem that women who take the POP have a slightly greater chance of developing non-cancerous (benign) ovarian cysts. These are not usually a problem; they are generally small, do not cause any symptoms and would not even be noticed. They are likely to disappear on their own. Occasionally, a larger one may develop, and may then cause some pain. I should stress that this is uncommon, and then stopping the POP normally makes the cyst disappear. However, if you have already had an ovarian cyst which needed treatment, then it seems sensible to avoid using the POP, as presumably you are already more likely to develop another one. You would be better off using a method which actually lowers the risk of an ovarian cyst, like the Combined Pill or injectable progestogens.

Ectopic pregnancy

One of the effects of progestogen is to slow down the movement of the egg as it goes from the ovary to the womb inside the fallopian tube. This means that, if a woman on the POP ovulated, and if a sperm had managed to break through the cervical mucus barrier, then it has very slightly more chance of meeting the egg within the tube. If fertilisation takes place, then an ectopic pregnancy (meaning a pregnancy in the wrong place) can occur. If it is not caught in time it can be dangerous.

You may have noticed the large number of 'ifs' in the last paragraph. An awful lot of things have to go wrong at the same time for a woman on the POP to develop an ectopic pregnancy, and since, after all, the failure rate is low, it is obvious they do not get the chance to go wrong very often. Also, of course, any woman can be unlucky and have an ectopic pregnancy, without taking the POP at all. The evidence for any effect of the POP is not conclusive, and there are a number of studies which do not show any increase in risk due to the POP.

In fact, some doctors would not even prevent a woman from taking the POP if she had had an ectopic pregnancy before (and was therefore known to be at higher risk of another one). I do not agree with this view: if you have already had an ectopic pregnancy, you do not want to place yourself at *any* greater risk, no matter how small, of having another one. You would be much better advised to use a method of contraception which actually decreases your risk, such as the Combined Pill or injectable progestogens.

However, if you have not had an ectopic pregnancy, then you should not let this possibility worry you in relation to taking the POP. Any increase in risk, if it does exist, is very, very small.

Other uncommon side effects

Very occasionally, women on the POP find they feel bloated (although they have not put on weight), or develop slight excess hair growth. These side effects are extremely unusual on the POP, as it is such a very low dose. Indeed, in my experience, some of these women find that there is no change at all when they stop, so the effect was probably not due to the POP at all. However, if this does happen to you, it is worth discussing it with your doctor. It is possible that these women might benefit if a POP was available which contained one of the new, more specific progestogens (see Chapter 3); unfortunately, this is likely to be a long time coming, mainly because the market at present is too small for it to be worth the investment on the part of the manufacturers.

HOW TO TAKE THE POP

If you are starting to take the POP for the first time, you should start your packet on the first day of your period, and you will be protected straight away. No additional precautions are required. If you are switching from the Combined Pill, finish your COC packet, and start your POP immediately, without having the usual seven-day break. Once again, no additional contraceptive precautions are required.

As I have mentioned before, the most important thing to remember if you decide to take the POP is to take it at the same time every day. You cannot afford to be more than three hours late taking this pill. In addition, you should take it every single day of the month – there is no stopping for periods as with the Combined Pill. In fact, many women find this an easier routine, as it is all too easy to forget to restart a packet after the break from the COC.

What do you do if you have taken a pill more than three hours late? Take it as soon as you realise what has happened, and then carry on taking your pills as usual. However, you will need to use additional precautions, like the sheath or diaphragm, for the next 48 hours. The same rule applies if you have missed a couple of pills – take the ones you missed, continue the packet, and use additional precautions for the next 48 hours. If, however, you forget your pill and have sex without using the sheath, then you should see your doctor for the 'morning after pill' (see Chapter 7).

These rules are not the same as the ones given by the manufacturers, and indeed, may not be the same as a leaflet you have at home. As more and more knowledge and experience has been built up about the POP, so it has become obvious that the rules in the past were far too strict. It used to be advised that you had to use additional precautions for 14 days if you missed a pill, as well as when you first started taking it. But if you remember that the cervical mucus effect wears off within 36 hours, it equally applies that it builds up again very rapidly. This is why a 48-hour rule is actually quite sufficient if you have missed a pill. Studies have shown that ovulation is extremely unlikely to happen before the seventh day of the cycle (day one is the first day of a period); by this time, both the cervical mucus effect and the thinning of the lining of the womb will have occurred. This is why no additional precautions are required when you start on the first day of your period.

Unfortunately, the wheels of science move far more quickly than those of bureaucracy. It takes a very long time for manufacturers to be able to change the instructions on their leaflets, as they have to go through a lengthy official procedure. And, of course, it takes time for other leaflets to be rewritten and published, with the added problem that there are likely to be copies of the old version still lying around. The result is that it is not unusual for there to be three quite different sets of instructions available at the same time – and then doctors are surprised that women are confused and make mistakes!

If you have had a baby

Although it is perfectly safe to start the POP immediately after you have had a baby, studies have shown that you are less likely to have problems with irregular bleeding if you wait for between four and six weeks after the birth. As I have already mentioned, the POP is safe to use during breastfeeding.

After a miscarriage or a termination of pregnancy

You can start the POP the next day, without the need for extra precautions.

ANTIBIOTICS AND THE POP

Although it is such a low dose, the POP is unaffected by many of the antibiotics which do affect the Combined Pill. The reason for this is based on the enterohepatic cycle, which I mentioned before, in Chapter 4.

After oestrogens and progestogens are absorbed through the stomach, they are transported to the liver, where they are partially broken down and combined with other substances. Some of these 'remains' are then sent back into the large bowel, from which they are in danger of disappearing altogether. However, in the large bowel there are a number of bacteria which are capable of converting the oestrogen products back into a usable form, which can be reabsorbed into the body and used. This means that the blood levels of oestrogen are 'boosted' by the hard work of these bacteria. However, the bacteria are not capable of producing useful progestogen products, so they have no effect on the blood levels of progestogen in the body.

When you take antibiotics, particularly the so-called 'broad spectrum' ones like penicillin and tetracyclines, they can temporarily wipe out these useful bacteria, and remove that extra source of oestrogen. This means that in some women, their blood levels of oestrogen can drop to 'dangerous' levels in that they might become pregnant. This is why additional precautions are advised if you take such antibiotics while you are on the Combined Pill. However, since the bacteria don't actually do anything useful to the progestogen, their disappearance makes no difference to blood levels of the POP user. For this reason, you do not need to use additional contraceptive precautions if you are given a course of antibiotics for cystitis, or a sore throat, or for acne.

There are, however, two antibiotics which will affect the POP, because they have an effect on the liver itself, speeding up and increasing the actual destruction of the progestogen by the liver enzymes. These are called Rifampicin and Griseofulvin. Rifampicin is used in the treatment of tuberculosis, but apart from that, you are very unlikely to come across either of these two.

THE ENTERO — HEPATIC CIRCULATION

O + P Metabolites

Oestrogen [Progestogen]

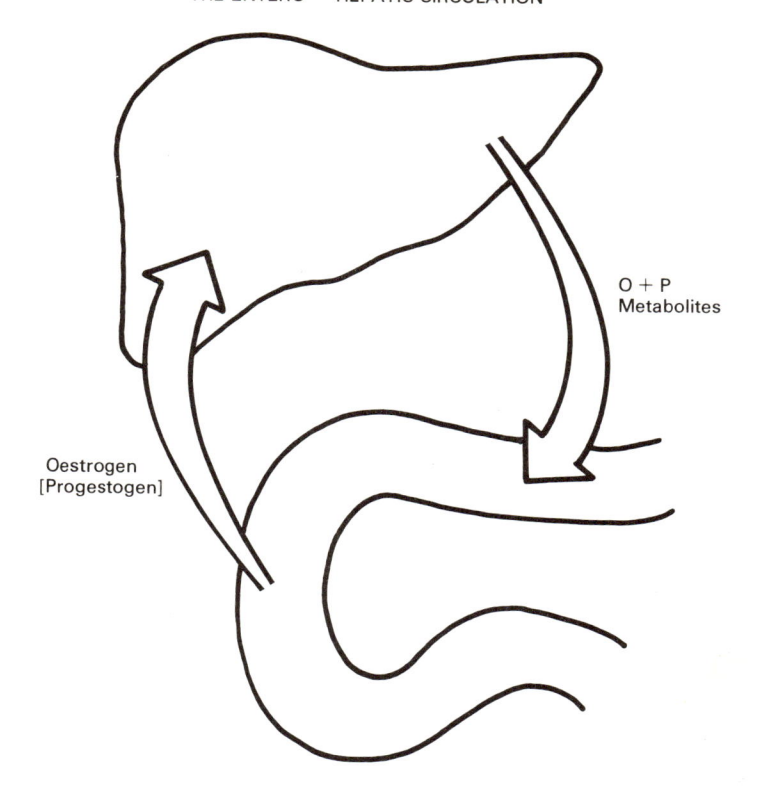

Figure 5.4 The enterohepatic cycle.

THE POP AND OTHER MEDICINES

Any medicines which speed up the work of the liver enzymes will decrease the effectiveness of the POP. This includes many of the medications used in the treatment of epilepsy (except sodium valproate or Epilim), Rifampicin as mentioned above and some medicines used in the treatment of mental disorders. A full list can be found on page 69, Chapter 4, as these medicines affect both the POP and the COC.

WHO SHOULD CONSIDER USING THE POP?

As you have seen in this chapter, the POP is suitable for almost everyone. It is probably best suited to women over 30, and to women who either cannot or do not want to take oestrogen. It requires good organisation to take the pills so regularly, but most women can cope in one way or another. It is an option which far too few women know about, but hopefully this is beginning to change.

6
INJECTABLE PROGESTOGENS

As their name implies, these consist of the hormone progestogen given in the form of an injection; they do not contain any oestrogen. This often leads to the mistaken idea that they must work and behave like the Progestogen-Only Pill (POP); however, although there are some similarities, there are also some very important differences.

HOW DO INJECTABLE PROGESTOGENS WORK?

In exactly the same way as the Combined Pill, by stopping ovulation 100 per cent of the time. This may seem surprising, when you remember that the POP is also a progestogen-only method, but has to rely quite heavily on making the cervical mucus impenetrable to sperm, as well as making the lining of the womb thin and hostile to implantation. Injectable progestogens do all that but, because they are also guaranteed to prevent ovulation, are much more effective. Indeed, their failure rate is only 0.1 per cent. This means that if 1000 women use this method for a year, only one would be expected to become pregnant.

Why are they so different? Well, the answer lies in the dose of progestogen used, which is much higher than in the POP. The graph overleaf shows the blood levels of an injectable and a POP over a period of three months. You will see that the dose of the injectable starts off high and gradually comes down, but is always above the level needed to prevent ovulation. The next injection is given before ovulation could occur. In contrast, the POP has much lower blood levels, which go up and down every day and cannot be relied upon to prevent ovulation.

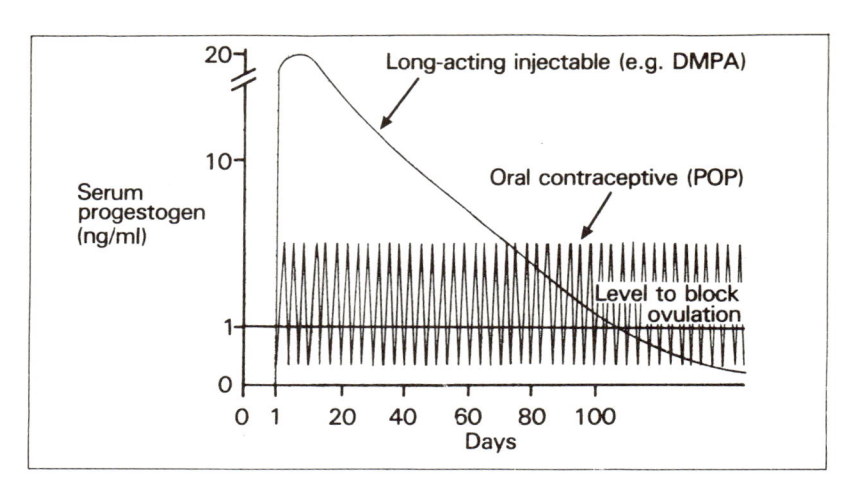

Figure 6.1 Comparison of the blood serum levels of progestogen in users of oral and injectable progestogens.
Source: modified from *Population Reports BS, Population Information Program*, John Hopkins University, Baltimore, USA.

Any substance which has to be taken by mouth is in danger of being destroyed by the stomach acids and enzymes, and, of course, will be affected by vomiting or diarrhoea. You would think that was quite enough of a hazard, but a hormone which manages to be absorbed into the circulation from the stomach can expect even worse dangers. The next port of call is the liver, which is ready and waiting to break it down as much as it possibly can. In fact, it is often quite remarkable that pills work at all.

A hormone given by injection, or by any route which does not involve the stomach, avoids all these problems. It is also less likely to be affected by other medicines, such as antibiotics, which can interfere both at the stomach and liver stages. And lastly, it is not dependent on a person with a less-than-perfect memory to remember to swallow it in the first place! All these factors combine to increase the efficacy and 'user friendliness' of injectables.

WHAT TYPES OF INJECTABLE ARE AVAILABLE?

There are two types on the market at present, called depomedroxyprogesterone acetate and noresthisterone oenanthate. I'm sure you won't mind if I refer to them by their brand names of

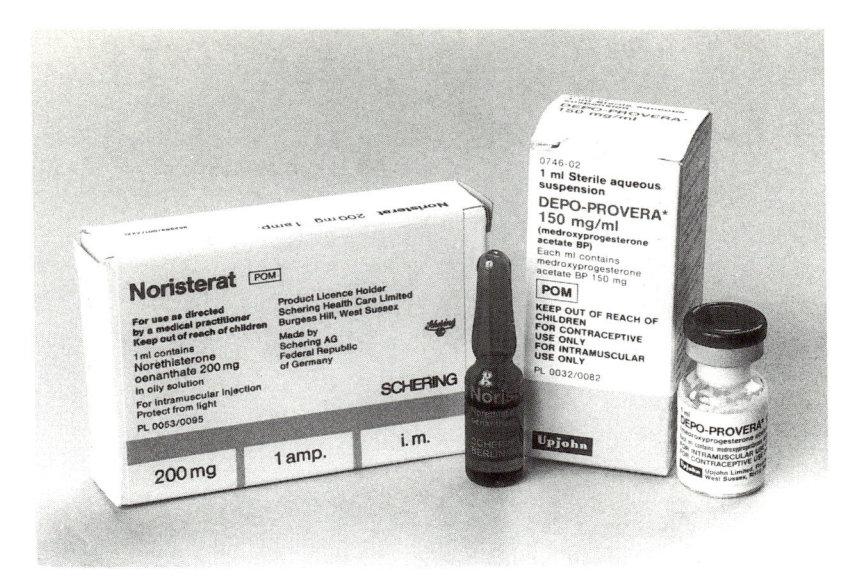

Figure 6.2 The two types of injectable progestogen currently available.

Depo Provera and Noristerat! The main difference between them is that Depo Provera is given every 12 weeks, while Noristerat is given every eight weeks. They are both intramuscular injections, which can be given either into the bottom or the upper arm. Noristerat, being oil-based, and therefore thicker, is a more painful injection, and is less used than Depo Provera. Since they are otherwise very similar, I shall refer to them collectively as Depo Provera, as what I say will apply to both.

THE ADVANTAGES OF INJECTABLE PROGESTOGENS

First and foremost, Depo Provera is an extremely effective method of contraception, free from the 'fear of forgetting' which is inherent in pill taking. Like all hormonal methods, it has the advantage of not requiring any special preparations for intercourse.

There are no oestrogen-related side effects or health risks. This means that it can be used by women who cannot take oestrogen, for example smokers over 35, and women with a history of problems related to oestrogen.

It is protective against pelvic inflammatory disease (salpingitis, or infection of the fallopian tubes) because of the cervical mucus effect. After all, if sperm cannot get through, neither will many bacteria.

Unlike the POP, but like the Combined Pill, it greatly lowers the risk of an ectopic pregnancy (a pregnancy in one of the tubes). The reason is the same: if you don't ovulate, there is no egg in the tube for the sperm to meet.

Similarly, like the Combined Pill, Depo Provera reduces the risk of an ovarian cyst. Again this is because it stops ovulation, thereby making the ovaries inactive.

For those women who suffer from sickle cell disease, it is now recommended as the best form of contraception. Users have been shown to have fewer relapses, or 'crises', and their blood shows an improvement compared with non-users.

If you have to take long-term medication which can interfere with both the Combined and Progestogen-only Pills, for example for the treatment of epilepsy or tuberculosis, you can still safely use Depo Provera. In this case, it is recommended that repeat injections are given two weeks earlier than usual. Similarly, if you are given antibiotics which interfere with either or both of the Pills, they will not interfere with Depo Provera, so no extra precautions will be needed.

Depo Provera can be used while breastfeeding, as it does not stop or reduce the production of milk. A small amount passes through into the breast milk, but no harmful effects have ever been found. It must be said, though, that provided you can remember to take it, the POP may be preferable; when combined with full breastfeeding, it is as effective as Depo Provera, and the dose is smaller, so even less passes into the milk. (Whether this is really important is debatable, but I am sure many women feel uneasy about even small amounts of hormone passing into their milk.)

The method is completely reversible, though there is often a delay in becoming pregnant. The majority of women will become pregnant between six months and a year after stopping, but this does mean that you need to plan a pregnancy about a year in advance. So you shouldn't start using it if you know you are going to want to become pregnant fairly soon. This delaying effect is the same whether you have had one injection or 50, so you should not worry that long-term use is likely to give greater problems.

If you are lucky, you will stop having periods, or only have them very infrequently. I have listed this as an advantage, since it really is one. There is no importance in having periods if you are not worrying about pregnancy, which you shouldn't be, while using Depo Provera. Indeed, if you think about it, it is *having* periods which is unnatural: in a society where there is no contraception, women are virtually always pregnant. You don't have periods when you are pregnant, nor, very often, while breastfeeding. So these women can go from one pregnancy to another without ever seeing a period. And, in fact, some types of cancer, for example breast cancer, cancer of the womb and cancer of the ovary, are much more common in women who have had many periods – those who started having periods very young, went through their menopause (change of life) late, and have had no children. I have mentioned this before, in connection with the Combined Pill (see page 20, Chapter 2), and it is just as applicable here. Indeed, it is thought that any method which prevents ovulation (and therefore periods) is likely to be protective against cancer of the womb and ovary, and possibly also breast cancer. Nor are periods necessary for 'purification'. When they don't happen, it is because the lining of the womb has become thin and contains few blood vessels. This is an effect of progestogen, which also helps prevent implantation. So there is no blood there in the first place – it doesn't build up, waiting to explode.

Having established that periods are unnecessary for a healthy life, think of the advantages; no worries about travelling, no period pains, no ruined underwear, no tampons, no imitation nappies.... Some women also experience an improvement in the symptoms of pre-menstrual syndrome, obviously, more so if they are not having periods at all.

Not everyone is so lucky, and you will find period problems also listed under 'disadvantages'. But, although you may start off with irregular periods, very many women find that their periods dwindle and stop completely by the end of the first year. Although textbooks say that the number of women having no periods at all is only 40 per cent by the end of a year, in practice this seems to be much higher. I imagine that for the purposes of research, even one day's bleeding in six months means that a woman cannot be said to have 'no periods' which will naturally lower the figures.

Depo Provera has no effect on blood clotting, so it can be used even by women who have had a thrombosis in a vein. It also has no effect on blood pressure. There is some controversy about its effect on HDL cholesterol levels; you may remember HDL cholesterol from the chapters on the Combined Pill. To briefly recap, HDL (high-density lipoprotein) cholesterol is good for your arteries, while other kinds of cholesterol are bad.

There have been a couple of studies showing that Depo Provera causes a slight rise in HDL cholesterol (i.e. good), a couple showing it causes a slight fall (i.e. bad), and another few showing it has no effect. All these studies have been quite small, and although they tell us little, do at least suggest that any effect it really has must be very minor, if it exists at all. Nevertheless, if you are already at very high risk of arterial disease for some other reason (for example, if you have a family history of lipid disorders), it would be best to discuss your case with a specialist, and probably have your blood levels of lipids checked before making a decision.

Despite 30 years of use, Depo Provera has not been proven to cause any kind of cancer in women. However, this area has been the subject of so much misinformation that I have devoted a separate section to it (see below).

DISADVANTAGES

Obviously, since Depo Provera is a long-acting injection, once given, you will have to put up with any side effects for the duration of its action (three months for Depo Provera, two for Noristerat). For this reason it is a decision you should think about carefully. In addition, you should remember that it may take a year to become pregnant after you stop. This is all very well if you can plan your life with some certainty, but is a disadvantage to those whose decision making cannot be so organised.

The most troublesome side effect of Depo Provera is undoubtedly the effect it can have on periods. I have already mentioned that many women will have infrequent periods, or stop altogether. However, before this happens (and for some women it never happens), you may get very irregular, unpredictable, possibly frequent bleeding or spotting. Indeed, before you make a decision to try Depo Provera, you should accept that this may happen to you, and that you could put up with it, at least for a few months, if it did. If you could not, for example because your religion would mean that your activities, both social and sexual, would have to be restricted, then you should not try this method. Equally, if you are about to go on a world tour, this is probably not the moment to try Depo Provera for the first time.

All is not lost if your periods are a problem. There are several ways of improving them: the next injection can be given a couple of weeks early, or, if you can take oestrogen, a short course of oestrogen may well solve the problem (often just one packet of the Combined Pill is used). And remember that with every injection, your chance of having infrequent or no periods get higher. So perseverance and patience are important, but therefore so is your conviction that this is the method you want to use.

Some women put on a few pounds when they start using this method, but the weight gain usually stabilises quite soon. Interestingly, women who are already overweight seem less likely to put on weight than women who are slim.

There have been some reports of women who are already prone to depression being made worse by Depo Provera. This type of side effect is very difficult to study, because depression is such a complicated problem and fluctuates over time. It does not seem to happen to women who are not normally depressed.

Since Depo Provera is a relatively high dose of progestogen given without any oestrogen, you would think that acne, greasy hair and loss of interest in sex would be a real problem. Surprisingly enough, although they do occasionally occur, they are uncommon. This is probably because Depo Provera has a different chemical derivation from most of the other progestogens in use.

DEPO PROVERA, CANCER, THE PRESS AND THE 'BAN THE JAB' MOVEMENT

Having read this far, you may have realised that Depo Provera really has a lot going for it. It is effective, has relatively few side effects and very few health risks. Why, then, haven't you heard of it before, or if you have, why was your impression a bad one? Why don't you know anyone who is using it?

To answer this question, we must look at the history of Depo Provera from the beginning. The first use of Depo Provera was in the mid-1950s, when it was given to women in very high doses both for the prevention of recurrent miscarriage, and also for a gynaecological condition known as endometriosis. Despite the fact that women were being given massive doses while they were actually pregnant, no ill effects were observed, and the United States Food and Drug Administration (FDA) approved it for general use in these conditions. In the early 1960s, it was noticed that women who had been given these large doses of Depo Provera during pregnancy did not seem to conceive for over a year after they had had their child, even though they were using no contraception. It was because of this observation, and because Depo Provera was already known to be safe, even in huge doses, that it was decided to try it as a contraceptive. This proved very successful, and an application was made to have it licensed for this use in the United States.

Just then, the results of some studies in beagle bitches were published. These showed that if you gave beagle bitches enormous doses of Depo Provera for several years, they would have a high chance of developing breast cancer. It says something about both the scientists and the self-image of the feminist movement at the time that it was immediately announced by the press that if it happened in female dogs, it would certainly happen in women. It was quite quickly shown that, in fact, beagle bitches had a natural tendency to develop breast cancer, with or without Depo Provera. Nevertheless, in the time between the first scare and its refutation, an enormous hate campaign against Depo Provera was started, which gained such momentum that scientific evidence became unimportant.

This 'Ban the Jab' movement resulted from a combination of worry about the health risks of Depo Provera, and the observation that it was being used primarily in developing countries. Campaigners thought that it was being tested on Third World women, who were uninformed about its risks, and who were being used as guinea pigs for the West.

At this point, it is important to understand that virtually all contraceptive methods are tested first in countries where the risk of death (both for mother and child) as a result of pregnancy is high. If you already had 10 children and knew that you had a very good chance of dying during your next (unplanned and unwanted) pregnancy, you too would be more likely to accept a small risk of side effects or health risks from a contraceptive method. However, in Western countries, the risk of dying as a result of pregnancy is very much smaller: thus, it is perfectly understandable that the acceptable level of health risks and side effects from contraceptive methods is lower. The balance of risks versus benefits is quite different in these two situations.

In fact, although it was (and still is) extremely popular in countries such as Thailand and Indonesia, Depo Provera was also being widely used in several countries, such as New Zealand and Australia, which might feel a little insulted to be thought underdeveloped and ignorant.

The campaign became increasingly heated, despite having less and less factual evidence on its side. The result was that, although the United States FDA had originally intended to

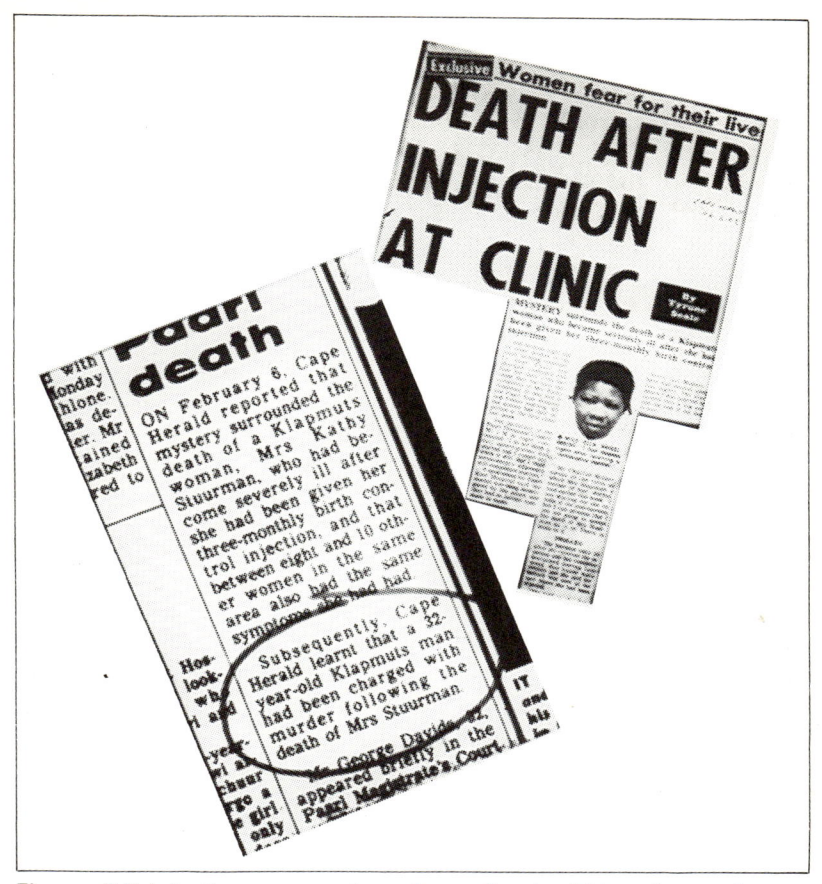

Figure 6.3 Injection scare story from South Africa. Later, it was discovered that the woman had been murdered.

license Depo Provera, political rather than scientific pressures forced it to withdraw its approval. Failure to be approved by the FDA is close to the kiss of death for any medication. All other countries look to it for guidance, and therefore become nervous of granting the product a licence themselves. Thus, Depo Provera was not licensed for use as a contraceptive in this country until 1984, and came in under a cloud of bad publicity. As you know, bad news always carries banner headlines, but good news is left to the last three lines on the back page.

In fact, the terms of the original licence in this country meant that its use was restricted to women who had had rubella vaccine, whose husbands were awaiting clearance after a vasectomy, or if all other methods were absolutely unacceptable. In practice, this meant that once again, Depo Provera gained a bad reputation as a method for those women who could not manage to use any other method, such as the mentally handicapped, the socially deprived and ethnic minorities. And, of course, if you read that it is a 'last resort' method, you are bound to look at it with suspicion.

Most doctors do not have time to keep themselves absolutely up to date with areas which are not their own specialty. As a result, there are still many doctors in this country who are worried about prescribing Depo Provera.

The reality of the situation is this: Depo Provera has been under study now for over 30 years, and has still not been proven to cause any kind of cancer in women. Long-term studies from many countries have shown no increase in the risk of breast cancer. However, a recent study from New Zealand, which showed no overall increase in the risk of breast cancer, did show a very slight increase in risk for women who had used the method for over six years under the age of 25. Needless to say, the number of women in this category was extremely small (less than 10) so this is not conclusive. It is interesting, though, that use under the age of 25 crops up here as well as in the studies on the Combined Pill and breast cancer. It has been suggested that perhaps this occurs because of the protective effect against benign breast lumps. Young women normally have lumpy breasts, which makes it more difficult to spot a cancerous lump, especially since cancer is so rare in this age group. If such a woman takes a hormone which 'smooths out' the benign lumps, the cancerous one will suddenly become more obvious. Thus, a woman who would have been found to have breast cancer several years later is diagnosed earlier, because of her choice of contraception. This 'unmasking' effect would explain the odd findings that, while Depo Provera appeared to slightly increase the risk in very young women, it also appeared to be slightly protective in older women. Although all this is very interesting, you should remember that the vast majority of the evidence is still in favour of there being no increase in the risk of breast cancer in women.

There have been a couple of poorly carried out studies which showed a slight increase in the risk of cervical cancer, but these are more than balanced out by eight other studies which showed no increase in risk, or indeed, a slight decrease in the risk.

It appears that, like the Combined Pill, Depo Provera has some protective effect against cancer of the womb (indeed, it is used actually to treat this cancer), and it is also likely that it offers some protection against cancer of the ovary.

STARTING AND CONTINUING INJECTABLES

Both Depo Provera and Noristerat should be given within the first three days of a period, and no additional precautions are then required. Thereafter, Depo Provera is given at 12-weekly intervals, and Noristerat is given at eight-weekly intervals. No extra precautions are needed either during stomach upsets or with most antibiotics, apart from those which speed up liver enzymes (see pages 67–9). If medication is used which does speed up liver enzymes, the injection interval should be shortened by two weeks.

WHO SHOULD CONSIDER USING INJECTABLES?

As you have seen in this chapter, there are many women who would find that Depo Provera is a very suitable method for them. Obviously, women who could not cope with any disturbance of their periods should not try it, nor should women who are likely to want to become pregnant fairly soon.

Although it has in the past been viewed with anxiety and suspicion, that is changing. More and more doctors have accepted that it is actually a relatively safe and effective method, and are moving away from the idea that it should only be used as a very last resort. And more and more women are realising that it gives them effective, hassle-free contraception. It can be very useful for professional women, especially those who travel and who therefore have to cope with not just a hectic schedule but also with time zone changes. Such women find the dual freedoms from pill taking and periods a blessing.

The most important thing about making a decision to use an injectable progestogen is that you should make an *informed* decision. Although this principle applies to every form of contraception, it is even more vital here, because you cannot change your mind for two or three months. In addition, you need to be prepared to put up with bleeding irregularities for a while, another decision you should have thought through beforehand. This chapter has given you the facts, but you need to apply them to your own individual case and then see whether it is really likely to be the method for you.

7

HORMONAL CONTRACEPTION AT SPECIAL TIMES

MORNING AFTER CONTRACEPTION

Although its name implies that you have to leap out of bed and rush to your doctor that same day, in fact, the most commonly used type of 'morning after pill' can be given up to 72 hours after the event.

The idea of trying to 'bolt the gate after the horse has flown' has been known since ancient times. Jumping several times immediately after sex was recommended, in an attempt to dislodge the sperm. Douching with various mixtures, some more revolting than others, has also been advised. All these methods are doomed to failure, because sperm can find their way into the womb within seconds of ejaculation.

Some effective way of preventing pregnancy after sex rather than before is clearly needed: young women having sex for the first time very often do not use any contraception, and do not have the courage (or the knowledge) to ask their boyfriends to do so. Couples using barrier methods of contraception, like the diaphragm or the sheath, are another major group in need of this service. Sheaths break, slip off, diaphragms are dislodged, or not used at all in the heat of the moment. And the last thing a woman who has been raped wants is a pregnancy by her attacker.

Various methods have been tried, mostly with high doses of oestrogens for several days, but these caused too many side effects. Nowadays, the accepted form of morning after pill is two high-dose Combined Pills, followed by another two 12 hours later. Nausea is a common side effect and about one-fifth

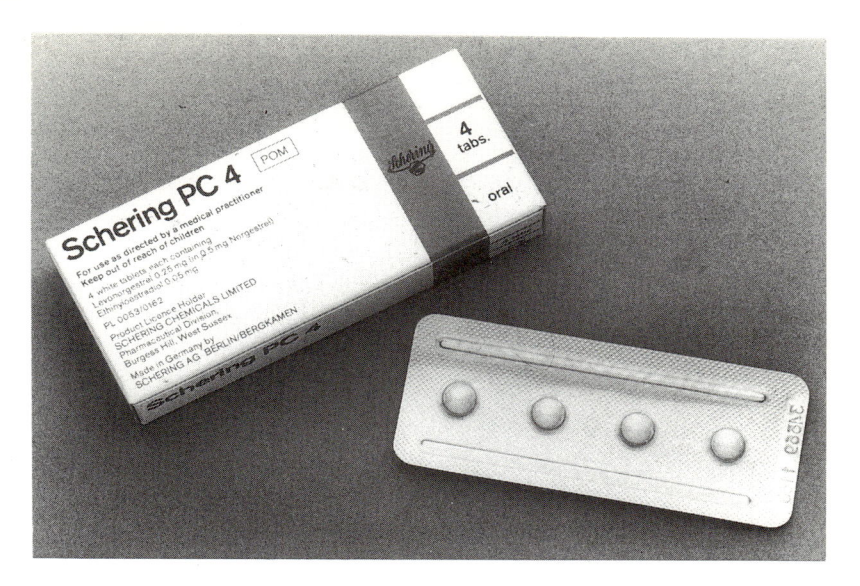

Figure 7.1 PC4 morning after pill.

of women vomit at some time during the 24 hours. If you do vomit within two hours of taking any of the tablets, you should go back to your doctor for more, as it cannot be guaranteed that they will already have been absorbed. It is not a bad idea to take an anti-emetic tablet about an hour before taking the pills to prevent vomiting – though this does make the whole thing rather more complicated, and, of course, anti-emetics can have side effects of their own.

As you can see, morning after pills are not an ideal form of contraception, which is why they are not recommended for frequent use. Quite apart from the side effects, you are taking such a high dose of hormones that you would be better off just taking the pill. However, as an emergency form of contraception it is clearly preferable to feel sick for a day than to be pregnant.

The morning after pill can only be used once in each cycle, after the *first* time unprotected sex has occurred. Women often think it is all right to have sex without contraception early on in the cycle, and then turn up for the morning after pill after sex on day 14. This is silly because it is perfectly possible to become pregnant as a result of sex as early as the fifth day: unfortunately, sperm can happily survive as long as seven days, so they can be sitting waiting for the egg when it appears. If you have had unprotected sex several times, or it is longer than 72 hours since it happened, you may be able to be fitted with an intrauterine device, which is very effective in this situation.

How does the morning after pill work?

It can work in two ways, depending on where you are in your cycle at the time. If you have not yet ovulated (released an egg), then it can work by delaying ovulation; hopefully, by the time you then ovulate, the sperm will have died. (Incidentally, you may now realise that it is very important that you use the sheath or diaphragm afterwards, since another, later arrival of sperm could still cause pregnancy.)

If you have already ovulated then it works by preventing the embedding of the fertilised egg in the womb (implantation). Some people object to this in the belief that this is an abortion, but this is not true. Abortion takes place *after* implantation has already occurred, while contraception is defined as the prevention of pregnancy *before* implantation. Indeed, if this were not the case, then both the Progestogen-Only Pill and the intrauterine device could be described as methods of abortion, since the POP (partly) and the IUD (mostly) rely on prevention of implantation as their method of action.

Will my next period come on time after the morning after pill?

As you may have already worked out, this must depend on when in your cycle it was given. If it is given before ovulation, and therefore delays it, your period is likely to be late. If it is given after ovulation then your period may be on time, or even early. In practice it is impossible to predict what is likely to happen in any individual case. Studies have shown that in the majority of women the next period comes roughly on time, while about a fifth have an early period and a tenth a late one.

How effective is morning after contraception?

In this case, effectiveness if quoted in terms of just one cycle, since this is the aim. In addition, the figures have to be adjusted for the fact that not everyone would have become pregnant anyway. It has been estimated that a woman has about a 30 per cent chance of becoming pregnant after just one act of unprotected sex mid-cycle. Based on this, the failure rate of the morning after pill has been calculated at between 2 and 4 per cent, the higher figure applying to mid-cycle (highest-risk) use. The intrauterine device is more effective, with only a few failures ever recorded. For this reason, if you need to be absolutely sure you will not become pregnant, you would be better advised to have an IUD fitted. However, IUDs have their own risks, so you should discuss all the pros and cons with your doctor.

Some women think that they will be better protected by the morning after pill if they take it within 24 hours, but there is no evidence to support this. The failure rates apply to use at any time within 72 hours. In fact, sometimes it is better to delay taking the first dose, for example if it would mean getting up in the middle of the night to take the second. Not only is it an unnecessary punishment to have to do that, but you might well sleep through your alarm and miss it altogether!

Can the morning after pill be used by women who cannot take the Combined Pill?

Usually the answer is yes. Remember, you are not putting yourself at risk of the long-term health risks of oestrogen, so, for example, age and smoking would not prevent its use. However, if you have already had a thrombosis (blood clot) then you should not take an oestrogen-containing morning after pill. You could still use an intrauterine device, or, if that was not possible or acceptable, a progestogen-only form can be used, but it has to be taken within 12 hours of the first unprotected sex in the cycle. This has a failure rate of about 3 per cent.

Are there any other health risks?

There is a very small possibility of an ectopic pregnancy (a pregnancy in the fallopian tube). This is very rare, but is one of the reasons why you are asked to come back for a check-up, just to make sure all is well.

If the method fails

Most women who use morning after contraception have done so because they really do not want a pregnancy at that time, and will therefore opt for termination if it fails. However, some women will not, and are often worried about the effect the hormones may have had on the baby. It should be said that if you know a termination would be out of the question, you would be better advised to use an intrauterine device rather than the morning after pill. Although there is no evidence that the baby would be in any way affected, this cannot be guaranteed. It is, however, reassuring that no cases of abnormality have ever been reported.

When should morning after contraception be considered?

- If no contraception was used. It is always worth checking

with your doctor, even if you think the risk of pregnancy is low – you might have miscalculated.
- Failure of a barrier method such as a sheath or diaphragm.
- Rape. You should also seek counselling and a check-up for infection.
- Forgetting to restart a packet of the Combined Pill. Most women think that the most dangerous pills to miss are the ones in the middle of the packet. This is not true. Once you have taken a week of pills, your ovaries are hibernating quietly, and it will take a lot to wake them. However, after your pill-free week, they have had seven days already without any pills, and may well be showing signs of activity. If you forget the first couple of pills of the next packet, you allow them to increase their activity to dangerous levels. In fact, 'let off the leash' they can actually be more active than usual, and ovulation could suddenly occur. If you have had sex without other precautions then you could become pregnant. So this is a situation in which you should see your doctor for the morning after pill and then you just continue with your packet as usual.

  If you forget pills at the end of a packet, the thing to do is just to restart the next packet seven days after the first pill you missed, i.e. to treat it as part of your pill-free week.
- If more than two Progestogen-Only Pills have been missed, and you have had sex without using additional precautions. Once again, you should see your doctor for the morning after pill and then continue with your packet as usual.

How do you go about requesting morning after contraception?

It can often be a problem, especially as the majority of 'accidents' happen at weekends. First of all, you need to check how much time you have, bearing in mind you have 72 hours for the morning after pill, but much longer (until five days after your predicted date of ovulation) to have an intrauterine device fitted. It is quite likely that you will have time to see your doctor in a clinic, even if it means waiting in the 'no appointments' queue. Many family planning clinics have an 'emergency' system, which allows you to come in without an appointment for the morning after pill. Some clinics (usually private ones) are open on Saturdays, so it is worth ringing round. Private clinics often advertise their services in women's magazines. If time is running out, and you see no way of finding a clinic, then you should call your GP (hopefully not in the middle of the night!) – it is, after all, an emergency. If you do not have a GP, the local hospital casualty department may be able to help, though please do not abuse their already overworked service.

Before you are given the morning after pill, the doctor should check that there are no reasons why you should not use it. You should discuss which method is likely to be most suitable for you, and any worries you may have. Also, if you have not been using any contraception, this is a good time to get yourself organised and discuss the options.

The doctor is likely to check your blood pressure, and may well do an internal vaginal examination. The purpose of the examination is to check that there is no abnormality present already which might confuse the issue later on if your period does not come, or if an ectopic pregnancy is suspected. You will be asked to return three weeks later to ensure that you have had a normal period, and that all is well.

If you decide to start either the Combined Pill or the Progestogen-Only Pill with your next period, you should start on the third day of your period rather than the first. This is so that you can be sure it is a normal period. You will still be protected immediately, without the need for extra precautions. Do make sure that you use some form of contraception until then, as you could still become pregnant as a result of unprotected sex after you have taken the morning after pill (see above).

HORMONAL CONTRACEPTION WHILE BREASTFEEDING

The Combined Pill should not be used while breastfeeding because it can stop the production of milk. However, the progestogen-only methods can all be used. The Progestogen-Only Pill (POP, see Chapter 5) is a good choice at this time, since it is more effective in combination with breastfeeding than it is on its own. In fact, in this situation its efficacy approaches 100 per cent. In addition, because it is such a low dose, and so little passes into the breast milk, it does not affect the baby. Indeed, it has been calculated that if a woman took the POP every day while breastfeeding for two years, at the end of that time, the baby would have absorbed the equivalent of just one tablet.

Injectable progestogens, such as Depo Provera (see Chapter 6), can also be used while breastfeeding. They also do not stop the production of milk, and there is no evidence that there is

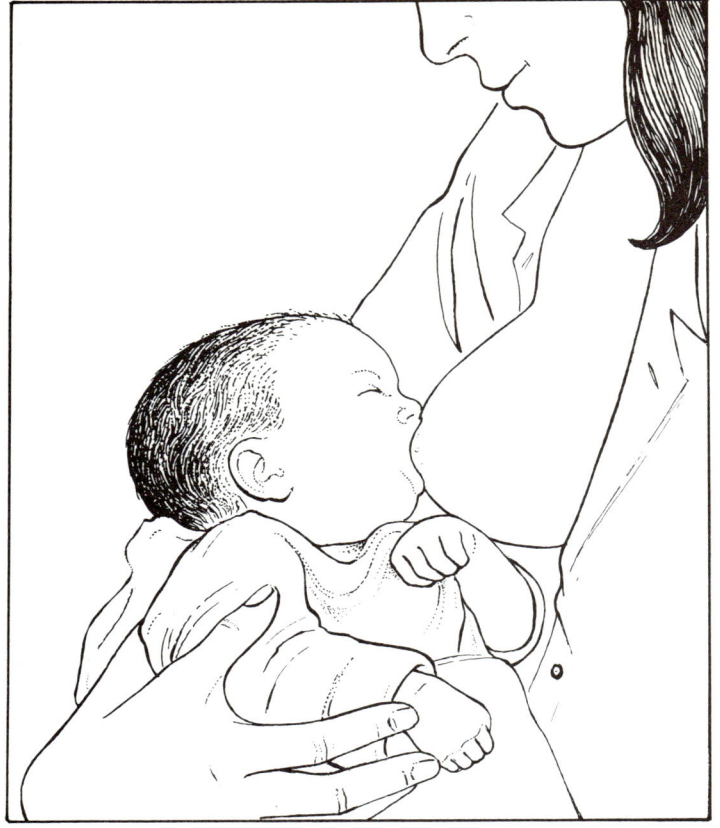

Maggie Raynor

Figure 7.2

any effect on the baby. Injectables have the advantage over the POP that they do not require you to remember to take pills. However, the POP may have at least a psychological advantage in this situation in that it is a lower dose, therefore correspondingly less must pass into the breast milk. Although there is no evidence that the higher amount from injectables has any effect on the baby, many women undoubtedly feel happier to know there is the least possible amount of hormone in the milk.

It is advisable to wait until the fourth or fifth week after delivery before starting either the POP or injectables. It seems that you are more likely to have irregular bleeding if you start earlier. There is no need to worry about other methods of contraception up until then, as ovulation has not been known to occur in a fully breastfeeding woman before the forty-third day after delivery.

The morning after pill is a problem while breastfeeding,

because the oestrogen could stop the production of milk, and, in addition, there is the worry of some oestrogen passing into the milk. The latter problem can be partly solved by expressing the milk for 48 hours and throwing it away. That does mean, though, that the baby will have to be bottle fed during that time, which may interfere with future breastfeeding. In general, the oestrogen-containing morning after pill is best avoided while breastfeeding. However, there are still two other options. There is a type of morning after contraception which contains only progestogen, though this has to be taken within 12 hours of sex. Its failure rate is normally about 3 per cent, though one might speculate that it could be more effective during breastfeeding (because breastfeeding in itself has a slight contraceptive effect). The other option would be to have an intrauterine device, which can be fitted up to five days after the predicted date of ovulation.

HORMONAL CONTRACEPTION FOR THE OLDER WOMAN

Don't skip this section, thinking it can't possibly apply to you: in gynaecological terms, you are an 'older' woman at 35! From the point of view of hormonal contraception, this age is also very important, since, if you smoke, you will no longer be able to use the Combined Pill.

It is ironic that women have until recently been denied oestrogen after the age of 40, even if they were non-smokers: this is precisely the time when their own ovaries are starting to slow down, their periods are starting to become irregular (often more frequent and heavier at first, and only becoming less frequent much later), and they start to get symptoms of the menopause, such as mood swings, depression, vaginal dryness and so on. This 'imminent menopause' stage can last several years and can be very distressing. Barrier methods of contraception, although usually effective at this age, will not relieve these symptoms, and women who have got used to the ease of the pill often do not make such a change easily at this time. And then, if you do manage to persuade a doctor to put you on hormone replacement therapy, it does not guarantee contraception.

The obvious solution to all these problems is to stay on the Combined Pill for as long as possible. And now, if you are a non-smoker who is generally healthy, you may well be able to stay on the Combined Pill until you are 50. This may sound

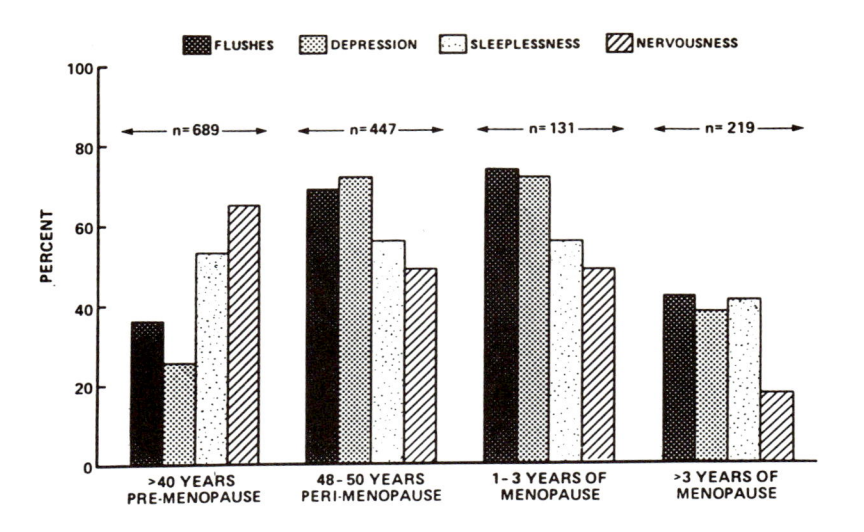

Figure 7.3 The incidence of symptoms of the menopause in pre-menopausal as well as menopausal women.
(Source: 'Hormone needs in pre-menopause' in *International Journal of Fertility* 30 (4) 1986, pp. 44–52 by G. Virginia Upton PhD from C. Lauritzen, 'The premenopause, in van Keep PA[1], Utian W.H., Vermeulen A. (eds): *The Controversial Climacteric*. Lancaster, MTP Press, 9, 1981.

incredible, but you should remember that the risks of the pill at this age (if you do not smoke) in the majority of cases will actually be less than those of pregnancy. Not only is pregnancy quite hazardous medically in the over-45s, both for the mother and the baby, but the psychological effects of an unwanted pregnancy at this time can be very severe. Indeed, in the United States, which is traditionally very conservative in its medical practices, the Food and Drug Administration's Fertility and Maternal Health Drugs Advisory Committee recommended in October 1989 that there should be no upper age limit for pill use by healthy non-smoking women.

This does not, of course, mean that doctors should be handing out the pill indiscriminately to women over 45. Your medical and family history should be taken into account; for example, if there is a strong family history of lipid- (blood fat-) related problems, it is likely that you will be advised to have a blood test to check that your blood fats are normal. Indeed, it could be argued that all women over 40 on the pill should have their blood fats and clotting factors checked. However, there is no evidence so far to suggest that this really would be useful for women who do not already have risk factors in their own or family history.

It is obvious that the lowest-possible-dose pill should be

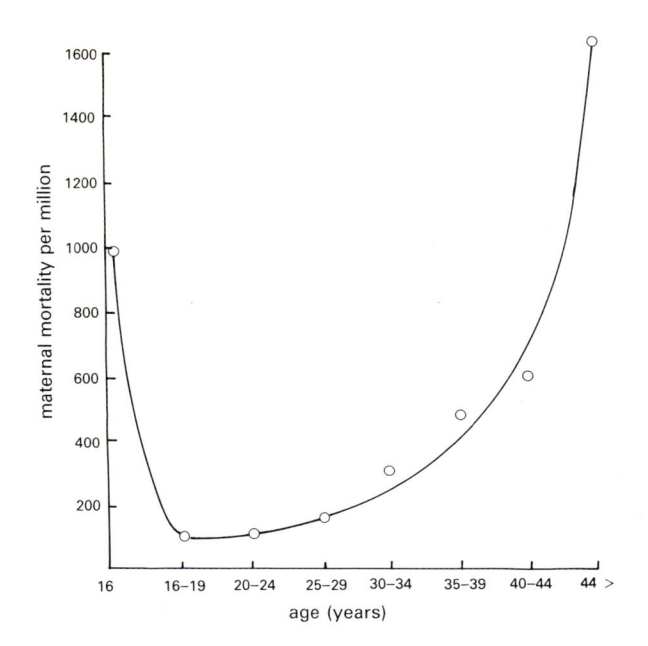

Figure 7.4 Maternal mortality per million births plotted against maternal age in years.

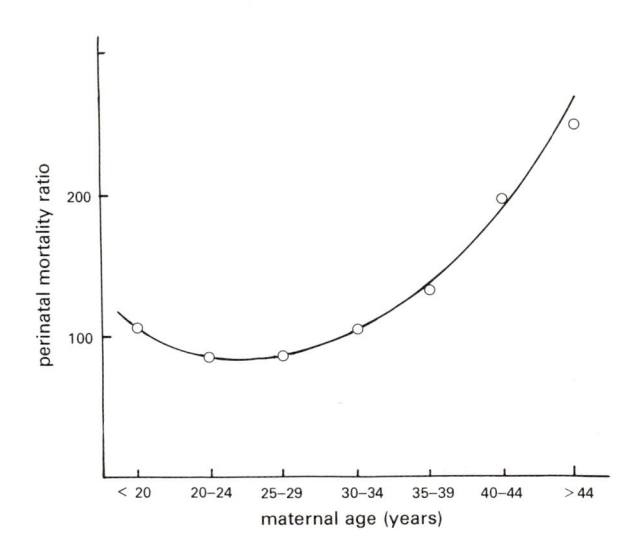

Figure 7.5 Perinatal mortality ratio plotted against maternal age in years.
(Source: Figures 7.4 and 7.5 from Beard, 1981, reproduced by kind permission of the Eugenics Society).

used, and that it should contain one of the new progestogens, to avoid problems with blood fats and sugars as much as possible (see Chapter 2). Mercilon seems the optimal choice at present, since it contains only 20 micrograms of oestrogen, combined with a new progestogen. Having said that, not all women are ideally suited to it, and any of the pills containing the new progestogens would be perfectly acceptable.

So here is yet another good reason to give up smoking! If you do not smoke, you may be able to stay on the Combined Pill till you are 50, and avoid all the problems of the 'pre-menopausal' years. At 50, you could change to the conventional type of hormone replacement therapy. A blood test can check whether you are actually going through the menopause; if it shows you are, then no contraception will be needed. If the blood test shows you might still ovulate, then usually a very simple method will offer enough protection, perhaps the sponge or spermicides alone. Fertility is very much reduced by this age, so methods which have an unacceptably high failure rate in young women are perfectly adequate here.

What happens if you smoke or have some other reason why you should not take oestrogen after the age of 35? Let me reassure you that there are solutions other than barrier methods or abstinence. Both the Progestogen-Only Pill (see Chapter 5) and injectable progestogens (see Chapter 6) can be used safely, even if you smoke. Injectables are extremely effective at any age, while the POP improves as you get older, so by the age of 35, the failure rate is about 1 per cent, and by 40 it is 0.5 per cent. In addition, most people become rather more settled and organised as they get older, so the three-hour pill taking rule for the POP is usually more manageable.

The real problems occur for those women who cannot take the Combined Pill, but who are getting menopausal symptoms in their forties. They need hormone replacement, but this will not provide the contraception which they also still require. This whole area can become quite silly, since it is quite possible to be taking more progestogen in hormone replacement than would have been contained in the Combined Pill! Also there are, as yet, no hormone replacements which use the new progestogens – so not only could you be taking more progestogen, but it may have a greater effect on your blood fats and sugars than one of the new generation Combined Pills.

Why take progestogen at all, when it is oestrogen your body needs? In fact, when hormone replacement therapy was first introduced, it did not contain any progestogen. Oestrogen on its own is actually protective against heart disease in menopausal women, and is usually well tolerated. It gives relief from hot flushes and other symptoms of the menopause, as well as quietly protecting your bones from osteoporosis (a process in which bone tissue is actually lost, making them weaker and therefore more likely to break). Unfortunately, with time, it was noticed that women taking it had a higher risk of developing cancer of the uterus (the body of the womb). For this reason, progestogen was added, and it has now been shown that it should be taken for 12 days each month to stop the increase in risk of uterine cancer. (The number of days for which it is taken appears to be even more important than the actual dose used.)

Adding progestogen introduced its own problems. For a start, it means that the woman is likely to bleed every month, a disadvantage to those who were glad to see the back of periods. It can also give annoying side effects, like headaches, but most importantly, it slightly increases the risk of heart disease. In practice, the increase in risk is cancelled out by the protective effect of the oestrogen – but you could equally say that the protective effect of the oestrogen is being cancelled out by the progestogen. Some doctors argue that the risk of cancer of the womb is extremely small by comparison with the risk of heart disease in this age group, and that it would actually do more good to go back to using oestrogen alone. The situation is still being argued fiercely within the medical profession, but at present the majority view is in favour of using progestogens.

Although there are no hard and fast rules about how to provide hormone replacement and contraception at the same time, there are some ways which have been tried and found successful. The basic idea is to take natural oestrogen (which affects clotting less than the synthetic type) and combine it with a progestogen. The oestrogen (which is usually oestradiol) can be given by mouth, but is normally given as an implant (a sort of glorified injection), which lasts three or six months. Then the woman can either take the Progestogen-Only Pill continuously, or take a progestogen for 12 days out of each 28. Using the POP can lead to irregular bleeding, while taking a (usually rather higher-dose) progestogen for 12 days each month will give a more regular bleed, but might give some side effects, like depression and headaches. In general, if you need this type of treatment, it is best to find a gynaecologist who has had experience in dealing with it, as he or she can advise you on what is likely to be most successful in your case.

I hope those of you who smoke will have realised that it might just be easier to give up the smoking than to have to stop the pill!

8

HORMONAL CONTRACEPTION IN THE FUTURE

The main feature common to most new methods of hormonal contraception currently being studied is that they are not designed to be swallowed. Any pill has to pass through both the stomach and the liver before it can start to work. This means that it will be affected by stomach upsets, or any condition affecting absorption from the stomach. In addition, while it travels through the liver, not only does the liver do its very best to destroy it, but, almost as if in retaliation, the oestrogen and progestogen affect other proteins and hormones which happen to be around. This war going on in the liver is called the 'first-pass effect', and results in both a weakening of the pill (which means you have to give a higher dose to compensate) and changes in blood clotting factors, lipids and various other substances; these changes are usually for the worse, so it would be nice if they did not have to occur.

Giving hormones by any non-oral route avoids both the stomach and the 'first pass' through the liver. This means that a lower dose can be given, since there does not have to be a 'reserve' to allow for loss through poor absorption or 'casualties' in the liver. Not surprisingly, a lower dose means fewer side effects and fewer health risks.

Unfortunately, all new methods of contraception take a very long time to reach the market. This is, of course, for your benefit, since the delay is mainly due to extensive monitoring and research to make sure they are not dangerous. Inevitably, most of them are made available first in the Third World, where the risk of dying due to pregnancy is so high that almost any method of preventing pregnancy is desirable. In developed countries, however, a woman is very unlikely to die as a result of pregnancy, so the risks of a contraceptive method become relatively greater. Having said that, the rate of approval (and to some extent, red tape) varies greatly from country to country, and some of the methods I am going to describe have been in use for several years already in European countries, while they are still waiting for approval in the UK. Spare a thought, however, for American women: they are always the last to get a new method of contraception, because the United States approval committee, the FDA, is extremely cautious, and they are also the first to lose it (because of the potentially enormous legal costs) if there is the slightest hint, even unsubstantiated, of a problem.

The majority of new methods do not contain oestrogen, i.e. they are progestogen-only methods. This partly reflects the anxieties about the Combined Pill in the early 1980s, since research is planned and started many years before anything actually appears for use in human beings. The more recent optimism has led to a renewal of interest in oestrogen-containing methods, but, of course, having been initiated later, these are going to take longer to reach the market.

It is very difficult to predict when a new method is actually going to be available: there are so many things which can cause delays, particularly unforeseen technical problems in manufacture. For this reason, I am only going to indicate broadly when you might expect to see each method – and I expect to be wrong at least half the time!

VAGINAL RINGS

Vaginal rings are in many ways the most exciting new development because they are so user-friendly. They are basically hollow, flexible, one-size rings which are inserted into the vagina and left there. They slowly release hormone, which is absorbed through the vaginal skin. They do not need any particular fitting technique, and they can easily be put in and taken out by the woman herself. This means that you have complete control over your method; you can remove it at any time.

There are several kinds of ring currently being studied. The one nearest the marketing stage is the progestogen-releasing vaginal ring.

This contains the progestogen, levonorgestrel encased in silastic. It is 5.5 cm in diameter and less than 1 cm thick. It is inserted into the vagina and left in place for three months. Like

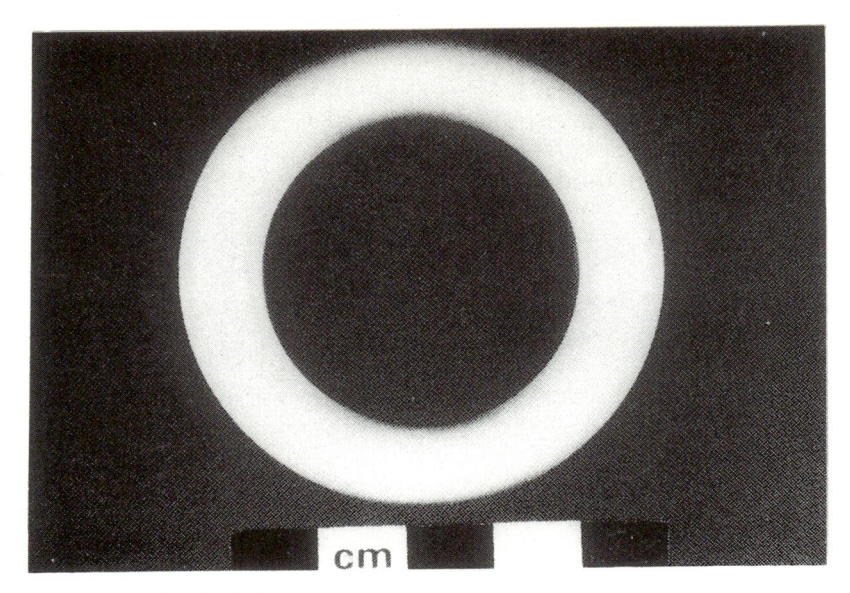

Figure 8.1 Vaginal ring.

the Progestogen-Only Pill (POP), it is not stopped for periods. However, it can be taken out for short periods of time, for example for cleaning, or even during intercourse. It is thought that it can be removed for up to 24 hours without any loss of efficacy.

It works in much the same way as the POP and therefore has a similar failure rate of three per 100 women years. Over half the women using it continue to ovulate normally, so, like the POP, it relies on making cervical mucus dense so that sperm cannot get through, and on making the lining of the womb thin and unlikely to permit implantation to take place.

Only 20 micrograms of levonorgestrel are released each day. This is a lower dose than in the POP – Microval, the levonorgestrel POP, contains 30 micrograms. As I mentioned earlier, avoiding the stomach and liver makes the use of a lower dose possible.

The main side effect is again similar to the POP, in that it causes irregular bleeding, especially in the first few months. This tends to settle down with time. Occasionally, the ring is expelled, especially if you have to strain when passing a motion, but then it can just be washed and reinserted.

This ring is effectively like taking the POP without having to remember to take pills – quite an advantage in view of the three-hour rule which is so important for the POP. And, of course, it has all the advantages of the POP in that there are no oestrogen-related side effects or health risks. It has proved extremely popular in studies in many countries, including the UK. Indeed, women in these trials often did not want to stop using it when the trial was over! So it looks as though it will be a very popular method when it becomes available, hopefully in 1991 or 1992.

Another progestogen-releasing vaginal ring is under trial, this time releasing desogestrel. Desogestrel is one of the newer, more specific progestogens, which have less effect on blood fats and sugars, and even fewer side effects, so this is a welcome development. However, it must be said that the dose used in rings is so small already that it is unlikely that it will have a major advantage in this respect over the levonorgestrel type. If anything, it is possible it may give slightly more regular bleeding, which would be an improvement. This one is at a very much earlier stage in development, so it is unlikely it will be available within the next ten years.

A ring releasing progesterone has been tried, for use during breastfeeding. The advantage of this would be that progesterone is a natural hormone (as opposed to the synthetic progestogens), and obviously, it would be better to use a natural version while breastfeeding if possible. Once again, this ring is still in early stages, and does seem to cause more bleeding problems than the others.

Combined oestrogen-progestogen rings are now being studied. A ring containing 15 micrograms of ethinyloestradiol and 120 micrograms of desogestrel has reached the furthest stage of development. This is a lower dose than the lowest-dose Combined Pill, Mercilon, which contains 20 micrograms of ethinyloestradiol and 150 micrograms of desogestrel.

This type of ring lasts for three months, but is taken out for seven days every three weeks to allow a withdrawal bleed, just like the pill-free week on the Combined Pill. It should give a regular bleeding pattern, also like the Combined Pill, but would have the advantage of being a lower dose, so there should be fewer side effects and health risks. Once again, this type of ring is unlikely to be available for some years.

IMPLANTS

Implants, as their name suggests, are placed or implanted under the skin, and slowly release hormone over long periods of time. At present, the types being studied contain only progestogen. The one which is most advanced in its development and research is called Norplant. Indeed, it is already available for normal use in many countries, including Finland and Sweden.

Norplant consists of six silastic capsules containing levonorgestrel. The capsules are 3.4 centimetres long and 2.4 millimetres thick. They are inserted under the skin usually of the upper arm through a very small incision, which does not require stitches. The capsules initially release between 50 and 80 micrograms of levonorgestrel every day and then the level slowly drops to 30 micrograms (the same dose as in the POP Microval). Norplant is effective within 24 hours of insertion and lasts for five years. The capsules then have to be removed through the original incision.

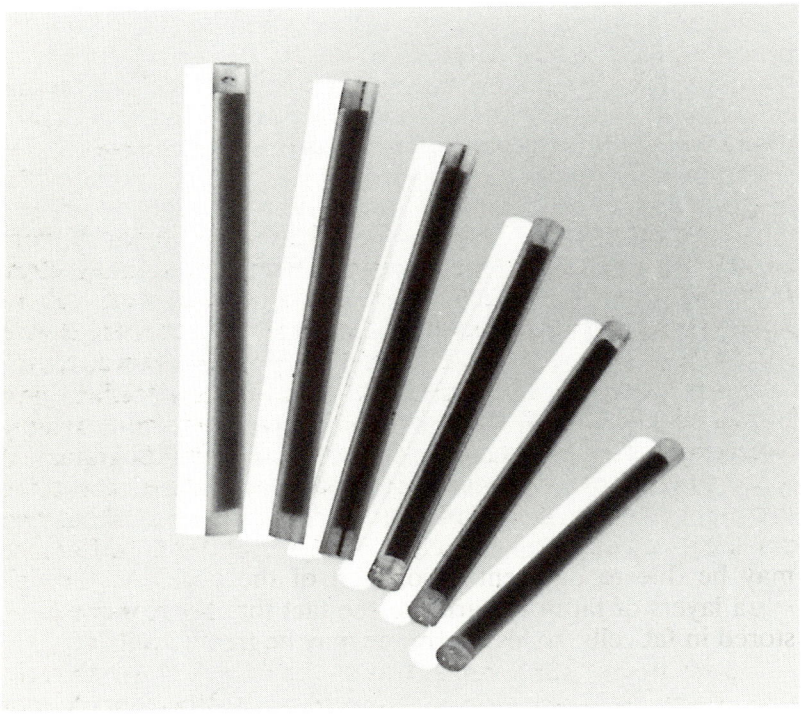

Figure 8.2 Six Norplant capsules.

(Reproduced by kind permission of Huhtamaki Oy Leiras of Finland)

The NORPLANT® Subdermal Contraceptive System

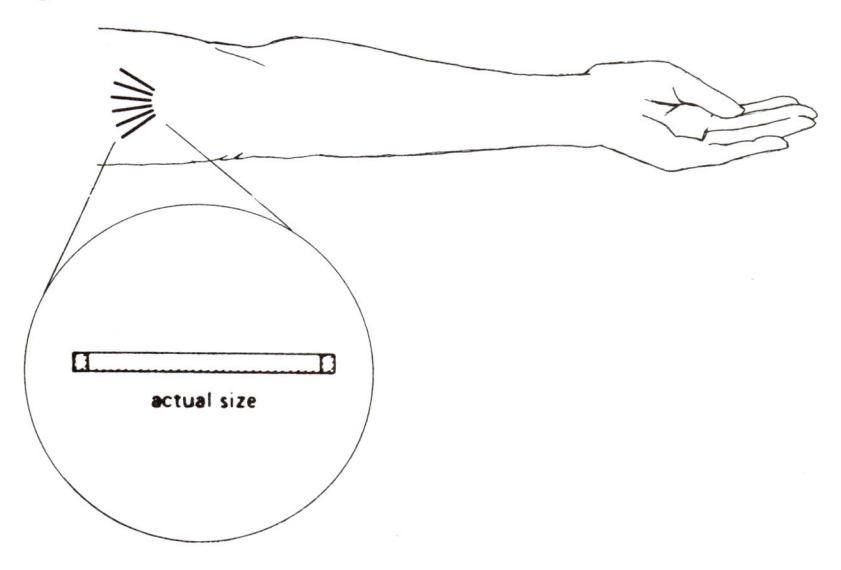

Figure 8.3 Where Norplant capsules are implanted in the arm.

The blood levels of Norplant (see Figure 8.3) are much more constant and steady than those of the POP, and it is therefore more effective. In addition, there is no need to worry about taking pills within three hours of the same time, as there is with the POP. The failure rate is about one per 100 women years, comparable to the Combined Pill. Interestingly, studies have shown higher failure rates in women who are considerably overweight. The important weight seems to be 70 kilograms – if a woman weighs this much or more, her failure rate using Norplant is doubled. (Mind you, that still makes it about two per 100 women years, which is pretty good.) The difference may be due to different absorption of the hormone through extra layers of fat in the arm, or the fact that hormones can be stored in fat cells, so less hormone may be freely available.

Norplant works in a similar way to the POP, but it is thought that a greater proportion of women using Norplant do not ovulate. It still needs to rely on increasing the density of the cervical mucus, to prevent sperm getting through, and on making the lining of the womb thin and unlikely to allow implantation to take place. Like the POP, because it contains no oestrogen, it does not have any oestrogen-related side effects or health risks. The dose of hormone used in Norplant is very small, and does not appear to have any effect on blood fats or sugars.

Once again, its main side effect is irregular bleeding, which tends to settle down after a few months. The other problem which sometimes occurs is infection at the insertion site: obviously it is important that a sterile technique is used, and keeping the insertion site dry for three days seems to help. This is a disadvantage of Norplant, in that it does need to be inserted by a trained person, and preferably in a clinic where sterile equipment is available.

An advantage of Norplant is that, although it lasts for five years, it can be removed at any time before that. The removal must be done by a trained person, so it is not as simple as the vaginal ring which you can remove yourself. Despite its long duration of action, there is no effect on fertility.

Six capsules are quite a large number to insert and remove, and it would obviously be better if the number could be

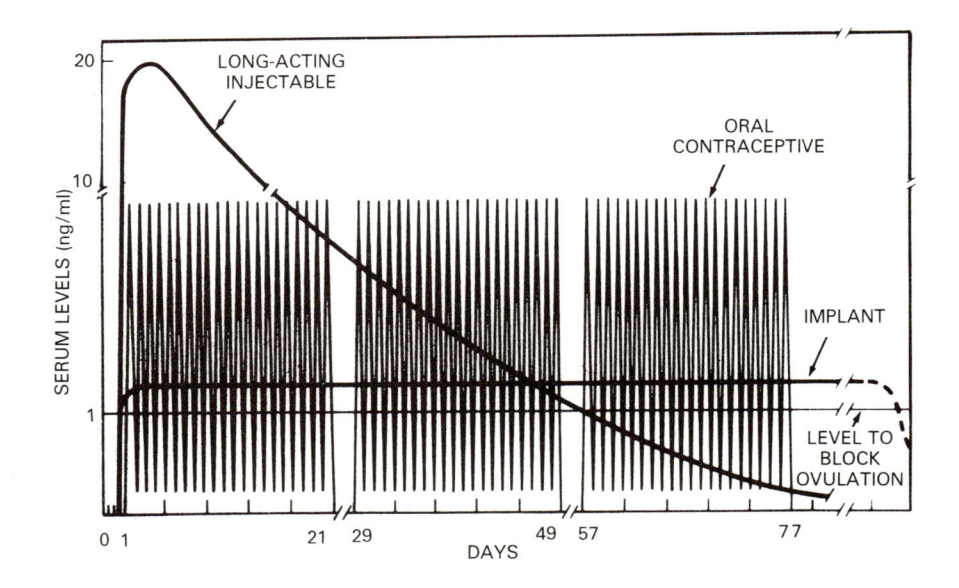

Figure 8.4 Comparison of blood serum levels of progestogen in users of Progestogen-Only Pills, long-acting injectable protestogens and protestogen implants.

reduced. The cosmetic appearance could also be improved: since the capsules are inserted immediately under the skin, they can be felt and sometimes seen. For this reason, a newer version of Norplant, called Norplant 2, only uses two capsules.

Norplant 2 is at an earlier stage of development, so it will not be available for some time. In addition, Norplant 2 has been held up by a problem with one of the polymers used in the silastic part of the capsules.

Norplant 2 lasts for about three years, a shorter time than Norplant. However, its easier insertion and removal will make it attractive for women who do not feel they need such a long duration of action.

Like the ring, Norplant and Norplant 2 have proved very popular whenever they have been used in research studies, and in the countries where they are available. They have the disadvantage, compared with rings, of requiring specialist insertion and removal, but they have the advantages of a longer duration of action, no involvement on the part of the woman, and a lower failure rate.

Since one of the problems with Norplant is its removal, research has been going on into biodegradable implants, i.e. ones which would just dissolve slowly by themselves and would not need to be removed. Of these, the one which may be available in the relatively near future is called Capronor.

Capronor consists of one capsule, similar in size to the ones used in Norplant, and which contains the same progestogen,

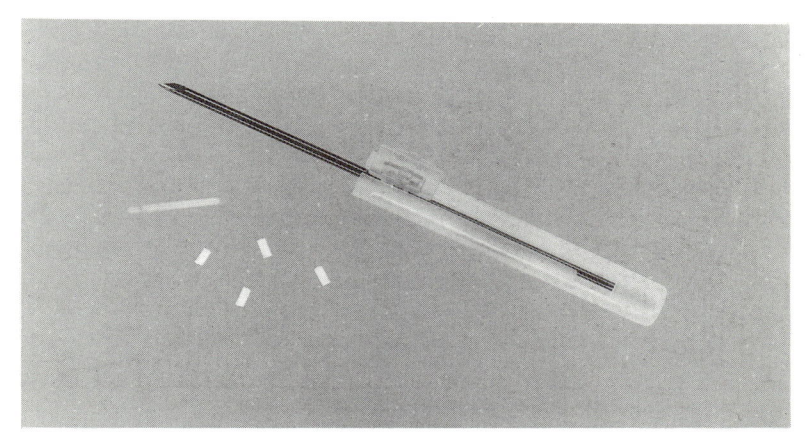

Figure 8.5 Capronor (long capsule at left) and contraceptive pellets are both long-acting implants that dissolve in body tissue and do not need to be removed. The special inserter can be used with either.

(Source: *Population Reports* from the John Hopkins University)

levonorgestrel. Once again, a small incision is needed to insert the capsules. Capronor provides contraception for about 18 to 24 months, and after that, the capsule is gradually absorbed.

There is another type of biodegradable implant which uses very tiny progestogen hormone-containing pellets. The advantage of these is that they are hardly visible at all. Four pellets have been found to give the best results, and give contraceptive protection for one year.

Although it may be an advantage to avoid having to remove the pellets, there is also a down side. Once the pellets have been put in, there is only a limited time during which they can be removed, so after that, the method becomes temporarily irreversible.

HORMONE-RELEASING INTRAUTERINE DEVICES (IUDs)

The idea of using IUDs as carriers for hormones is not a new one. Indeed, for some years already a progesterone-releasing IUD, called the Progestasert, has been available. However, this particular type has been almost completely abandoned because it caused a great deal of irregular bleeding and spotting, and, more importantly, it had a higher than average rate of ectopic pregnancies (pregnancy outside the womb, usually in the fallopian tube). Since the risk of an ectopic pregnancy is already relatively high with an ordinary IUD, an increase was obviously unacceptable.

For some years now, researchers have been looking at a different kind of IUD, which releases levonorgestrel. This type of IUD seems to be quite remarkable. Instead of increasing the risk of an ectopic pregnancy, it actually reduces it to below normal levels. And whereas IUD use is normally associated with an increased risk of developing pelvic inflammatory disease or salpingitis, this type again reduces the risk. The list of wonders goes on. Normally, IUD use leads to heavier and more painful periods: although some spotting does occur with the levonorgestrel-releasing device, periods are much lighter and less painful.

So this IUD has overturned all the side effects normally associated with IUDs, and, in addition, is more effective, with a failure rate of about one per 100 women years.

It has been suggested that this might be the ideal method of contraception for the woman who needs contraception as well as hormone replacement therapy. One of the problems with hormone replacement therapy is that the only hormone which it is really necessary to replace is oestrogen. Unfortunately, progestogen has to be given as well because it has been shown that if oestrogen is given on its own, the woman is at higher risk of developing cancer of the womb. As given at present, by mouth and for about 12 days each month, the progestogen can lead to side effects, such as headaches and depression. All that could be changed if the woman took oestrogen alone as her hormone replacement therapy, and had a progestogen-releasing IUD to give both contraception and protection against cancer of the womb at the same time. There is also a good chance, in these circumstances, that she would not have periods at all, something which the majority of women using hormone replacement therapy welcome.

Technical problems have so far delayed the production of the levonorgestrel-releasing IUD, but meanwhile, a desogestrel-releasing version has appeared on the scene. This will, of course, require many years of research, but may be an improvement, because of the newer, more specific type of progestogen.

OTHER POSSIBILITIES FOR THE MORE DISTANT FUTURE

Here I am going to mention briefly some ideas which are still at an early stage of development. Having said that, some are more advanced than others, and one can never tell when a breakthrough will occur which leads to a method suddenly becoming viable much more quickly.

In Chapter 6, I discussed the many advantages of injectable contraceptives, such as Depo Provera. The main problem with this type of contraception is irregular bleeding. Attempts at improving this are being made all the time, and one of the more promising is Cyclo Provera, which is a monthly injection of 25 mg of Depo Provera plus 5 mg of oestradiol cypionate. Of course, this is no longer a progestogen-only method, since it does contain oestrogen, and therefore may cause some oestrogenic side effects and health risks. However, like Depo Provera, it removes the need to remember to take pills, and avoids the stomach and liver. In addition, it does give quite regular cycles, and, being only monthly, can be stopped more quickly than Depo Provera.

The possibility of a 'unisex' pill, which could be used by both men and women, is certainly novel and appealing. This method is based on the use of a hormone called 'inhibin'. It appears to be important in both men and women, in the production of sperm and eggs. It is thought that if artificially high doses of it were given, it would halt the production of eggs in women and sperm in men, and, because it does not seem to have any other action, there should be very few side effects.

A few years ago, there was great enthusiasm about a nasal spray contraceptive. This works by stopping ovulation, like the Combined Pill, but does it at an earlier stage in the process. Very low levels of the hormone used are needed, and it is given as a spray because it is very well absorbed through the nasal skin, thus also avoiding the stomach, where it would be completely destroyed. Unfortunately, because it does not replace the oestrogen which it stops from being produced, it induces a menopause, complete with hot flushes. Obviously, this is unacceptable, and so the scientists have had to go back to the drawing board and think of ways of preventing this from happening.

Patches are all the rage in the world of hormone replacement therapy at the moment. A patch is simply like a sticking plaster which contains hormone. The patch is stuck on the skin, and the hormone is gradually absorbed through the skin, once again (this is beginning to be very repetitive . . .) avoiding the stomach and liver. People can have an allergy to sticking plaster, and so some women do develop a reaction to the hormone patches, but otherwise they are generally very popular. So far, it has proved fairly simple to give oestrogen via a patch, but it seems to be more difficult to combine it with progestogen. Nevertheless, once this problem is overcome, it should be possible to use patches for contraception, thereby avoiding the use of pills, and the trauma of injections or implants. Of course, the patches would probably have to be replaced every couple of days, so it would involve a certain amount of remembering on the part of the woman, which is a disadvantage. Nevertheless, this would almost certainly be a popular method if it became available.

In general, it is not advisable to become overenthusiastic about any new method until it actually reaches the market. There are so many possible disasters along the way – a new side effect or health risk becomes suddenly apparent, the material used to hold the hormone is found to be dangerous or unstable, the company discovers something else which they find more exciting and simply stops putting money into the older product – these are just a few. Nevertheless, it is good to know that research is going on, since none of the methods we have at present could be described as 'perfect' by a long way. Complacency should be avoided in any branch of medicine.

9

HORMONAL CONTRACEPTION FOR MEN

There can be few areas in contraception where so much has been discussed and so little delivered. The 'male pill' has been awaited for decades, but seems no nearer now than 20 years ago. Why?

Well, first of all, we should consider the attitudes which prevailed then and are still around now. 'Who needs a male pill anyway? Contraception is the woman's responsibility.' And then, would you trust a man who said, 'It's all right, darling, I'm on the pill'?

Whereas the first statement is clearly untrue, the second point is very pertinent. Many women find it difficult to remember to take their pill, even with the best intentions – and they are in a position where they may suffer for their poor memory by becoming pregnant. If a male pill was available, how could you be sure the man had taken it? There would always be men who would lie. And even among those who were genuinely trying, how could you guarantee they had not forgotten, when they would not be living in fear of pregnancy? This is actually rather well illustrated by a poster which has been used to try and increase men's involvement in contraception, shown overleaf.

Having said all that, there is clearly a need for a male contraceptive, which would probably be used mainly in stable, long-term relationships. Such couples could then share the responsibility for contraception. This attitude can already be seen in the growing numbers of men who have vasectomies, a frequent comment being 'It's my turn now'.

Unfortunately, research into contraception has tended to

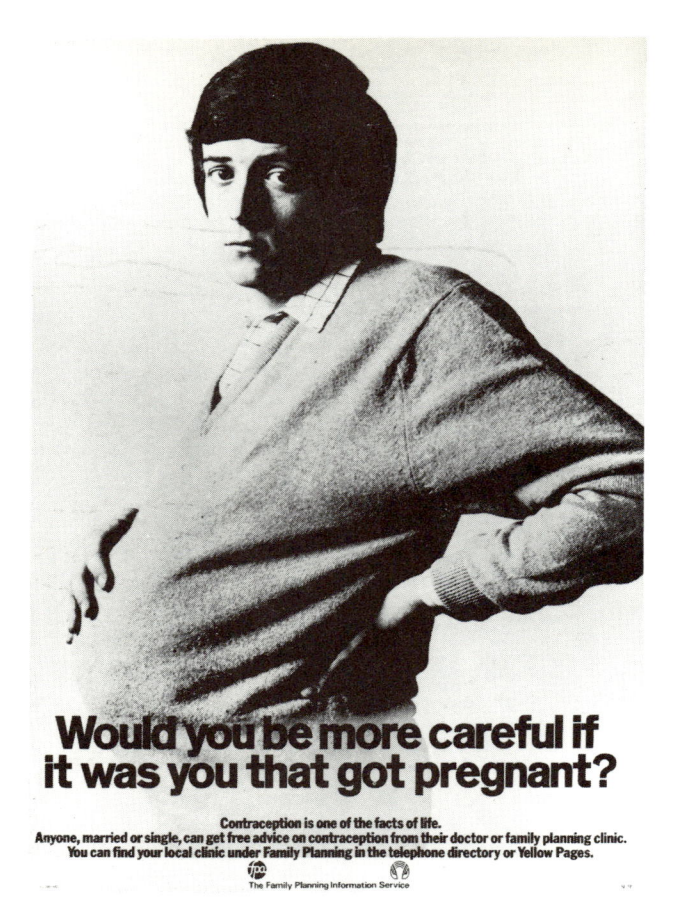

Figure 9.1 Family Planning Association campaign poster (reproduced by kind permission of FPA).

focus on female methods. It has been estimated that only about 8 per cent of the money spent on contraceptive research throughout the world has been targeted at the development of male contraceptives.

Lack of money has been compounded by the practical difficulties of developing a contraceptive for men. To understand why, we must briefly look at the reproductive process in men.

The whole system is governed by a hormone called Luteinising Hormone Releasing Hormone (LHRH) or Gonadotrophin Releasing Hormone (GnRH). These are two names for the same thing, and I shall refer to it as GnRH to try and avoid confusion. GnRH is produced by the hypothalamus, an area in the brain, and goes to the pituitary gland, also in the brain.

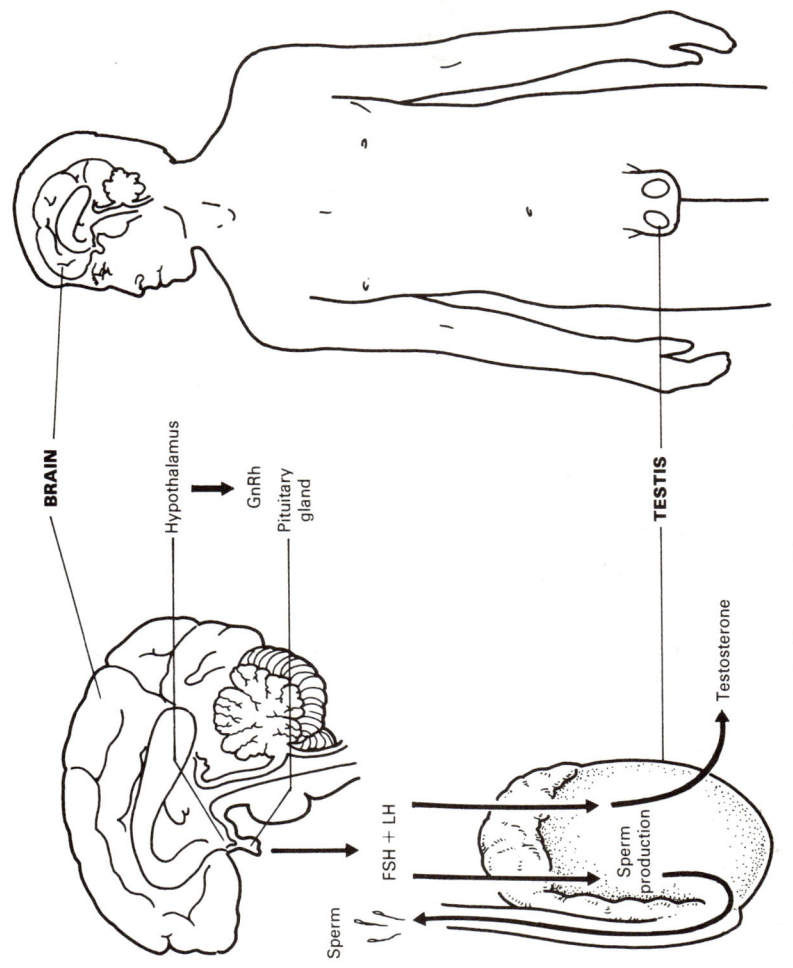

Figure 9.2 The release and effects of hormones in men.

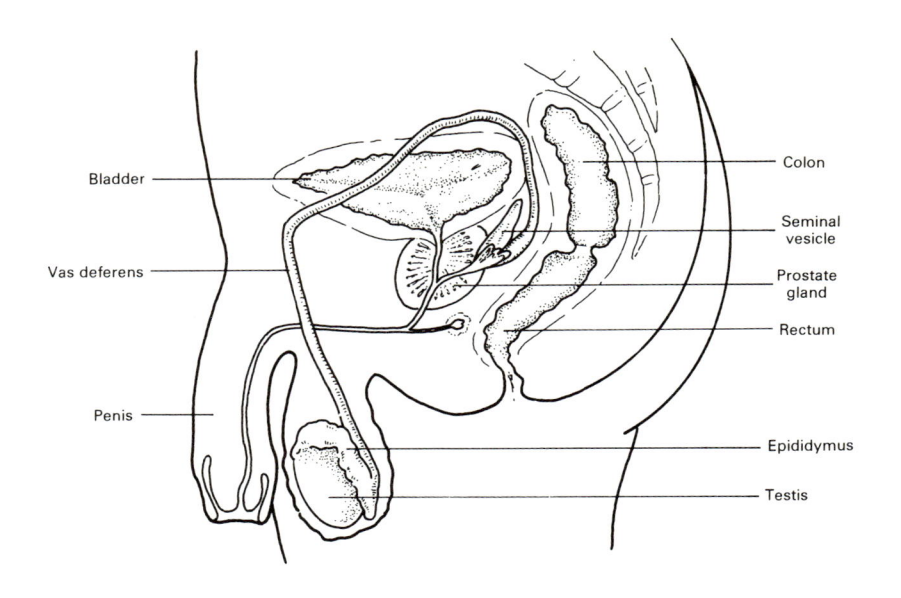

Figure 9.3 Male reproductive organs.

Once there, it stimulates the production of two hormones, Follicle Stimulating Hormone (FSH) and Luteinising Hormone (LH). These two hormones, FSH and LH, both disappear off to the testes in the bloodstream and influence events there. FSH is responsible for the formation of sperm themselves, while LH makes the testis produce another hormone, testosterone. Testosterone is responsible for making men look like men and for male libido (sex drive). So FSH makes sure the sperm are ready and waiting, while LH and testosterone make the man want to do something about it.

Sperm spend about three months sitting around in the testis before they are ready to leave for the outside world. They have to move around nearly a mile of small tubes, finally reaching the epididymis, where they rest for about 12 days, and then into the vas deferens, which enters the penis. Even then, they are not completely 'finished'; they only become fully active once they find themselves in the woman's vagina.

You would think that with so many stages in their production, it would be relatively simple to block one at least. Unfortunately, there are several problems, not the least of which is the sheer number of sperm being produced – 100,000 *per minute*. I leave you to calculate how many must be present after three months: I promise you it is a very, very large number. And it's not just a case of 'well, let's kill or prevent as many as possible', because you only have to have *one* persistent little sperm to cause a pregnancy. It sheds new light on the phrase 'safety in numbers'.... Although men who are considered infertile often have what is called a 'low sperm count' rather than no sperm at all, their sperm are usually also not very mobile or active, so that fertilisation does not occur. However, in an otherwise fertile man, the presence of a 'low sperm count' can still easily lead to pregnancy.

Another major problem is that you will notice that there is really quite a fine dividing line between the hormones responsible for sperm production and sex drive (FSH and LH). It is all too easy to stop the man being interested in (and therefore capable of) sex, in which case the contraceptive properties of the drug become rather academic.

The other problem is that many methods will take three months to become effective, because of the large store of sperm already present. This means there has to be a period of waiting, during which some other method of contraception must be used. Equally, it may take three months for the sperm store to build up again after the contraceptive is discontinued, prolonging the wait for a desired pregnancy.

Anxieties do not stop there. If you mess around with the production of sperm, how do you know that abnormal ones will not be produced, leading to abnormal babies? This could happen at any time, but particularly during the first few months while the contraceptive effect is not absolute, and during the few months after stopping, when sperm are beginning to reappear. The same argument holds if you try and alter sperm to make them inactive: you have to be sure that there is no halfway stage, where they could still lead to pregnancy, but are abnormal.

As mentioned above, there are two main options in male contraception: firstly, to try and stop the production of sperm, and secondly, to try and inactivate the sperm after they have been produced. Let us consider each of these options in turn.

METHODS WHICH ATTEMPT TO STOP THE PRODUCTION OF SPERM

Look again at the drawing on page 125. You will see that there are several possible times to interfere with the process of sperm production. The obvious place to start is at the hypothalamus.

If the production of GnRH is completely stopped, nothing else will happen. Unfortunately, *nothing* else will happen. Remember that GnRH is also responsible for the production of LH, which gives men their sex drive, so the man will become impotent. Clearly, this is unacceptable, so if this approach is to be used, the man must be given some testosterone as compensation. Anti-GnRH products cannot be given by mouth, as they are rapidly destroyed in the stomach, so methods such as nasal sprays have been developed. However, this is very expensive, and when you add the cost and complexity of giving testosterone at the same time, it all becomes very costly and cumbersome. Side effects are also a nuisance: for example, men given GnRH blockers can develop hot flushes, rather like the female menopause. All in all, this does not look like a very promising approach.

The other way of trying to reduce (rather than completely stop) the production of GnRH is to flood the body with steroids. You could actually give men the female contraceptive pill, but its effectiveness is counterbalanced by the fact that they start to change into women....

One of the most promising ideas is to give Depo Provera together with testosterone as monthly injections. This both reduces GnRH production, and provides 'hormone replacement' via the testosterone. Monthly injections are not much fun, however, and may not be acceptable to many men, even though the method appears to be reasonably effective.

In order to try and overcome this problem, and make the method a self-administered one, oral medroxyprogesterone has been tried, combined with testosterone cream (testosterone cannot be given by mouth as it is rapidly destroyed in the stomach). Apart from reduced efficacy, this method had an unexpected side effect: the women partners of these men started to grow moustaches and have excess hair generally! It turned out that they were absorbing some of the testosterone cream which remained in their partner's skin and was transmitted in sweat.

Testosterone by itself has been tried, but has to be given by weekly injections. It does not seem to cause a complete halt in sperm production, which is a problem. As mentioned earlier, this really has to be an all or nothing approach, since only a single healthy sperm is needed to cause pregnancy.

A variant of testosterone, called 19-nortestosterone, may be more promising in that it is stronger and therefore lasts longer. Nevertheless, this is still in the early stages of investigation.

Let us move down now to the pituitary gland. This is where

the hormones FSH and LH are produced. The important thing here is to halt the production of FSH while leaving LH alone. There seem to be two possible ways of doing this.

The first is a remarkable hormone called inhibin. Scientists were predicting the existence of this hormone some 60 years before it was actually discovered. Inhibin is produced by the testis and specifically inhibits the production of FSH. It has no effect on LH, and therefore does exactly what is wanted: it stops the production of sperm without any effect on sex drive. In fact, it has also been considered for use in women, in whom it also has a very specific action in preventing ovulation. For this reason, it is sometimes referred to as the 'unisex' pill. But don't get too excited yet. It turns out that inhibin is an incredibly complicated molecule (or rather two molecules, which do not necessarily have the same effects when separated), and is keeping scientists very busy trying to synthesise it. It is all very well finding it in its natural state in the testis, but unless it can be made synthetically in a laboratory, it is quite impractical for production as a widely used contraceptive. This process is extremely expensive and time-consuming, so although it seems very exciting, it is still a long way off.

The other way to attack FSH specifically is to try and produce a vaccine against it. Although this seems very logical, it has many problems. For a start, different individuals have different responses to a vaccine, and so some men would need boosters much sooner than others. It is not very practical to have to continually monitor one's sperm count. In addition, the vaccine itself causes quite a nasty local reaction in the skin, and ulcers have been known to form. This is clearly unacceptable, especially when you think that it is not even a dangerous 'disease' that the man is being vaccinated against!

METHODS WHICH ACT DIRECTLY AGAINST SPERM PRODUCTION IN THE TESTIS ITSELF

The problem with drugs which effectively poison the cells producing sperm in the testis is that they tend to poison the man as well. This is an unfortunate side effect, which has rather put a damper on this type of research.

The most famous of these compounds is a drug called gossypol, which was discovered in China quite by chance. It was noticed that in one particular rural area of China, the men seemed to be much more likely to be infertile. This was a cotton-growing area, and it was eventually discovered that the crucial factor was that they were frying their food in cotton seed oil. China has a rather large overpopulation problem and so they got very excited and started doing large trials giving gossypol to men. It certainly proved very effective – so much so that about 10 per cent of the men became infertile for ever. In addition, gossypol has the effect of lowering the amount of potassium in the body: this at first results in the man feeling tired and weak, but can eventually lead to complete muscle paralysis (including the heart ...). So gossypol is not the answer after all, but there is considerable interest in producing a derivative of it which might be an effective, reversible contraceptive without the side effects.

Desperation seems to be a good catalyst for new research ideas, and so China has come up with another drug which they hope will be more acceptable than gossypol. This is an extract of the Thunder God vine, used in traditional Chinese medicines for many years. It was noticed that men given medicine containing this extract seemed to be more likely to be infertile, and did not appear to get other side effects. Trials are going on in China, and the rest of the world is watching with interest.

METHODS WHICH TRY AND STOP THE MATURATION OF SPERM IN THE TESTIS

Certain sugars seem to be necessary for the well-being of sperm while they sit in the epididymis, and so producing substitutes which are very similar, but block rather than help sperm metabolism, have been tried. The advantage of this approach is that it would be effective very rapidly (within a few days) as opposed to the three months normally required. So far, they seem to produce side effects in the nervous system, which limits their potential.

A rather notorious example of this approach is cyproterone acetate, an anti-androgen which seems to affect the function of sperm which are in the epididymis. This drug became infamous after it was used in high security prisons to reduce the sex drive of inmates. Because of its effects on libido, it is not a viable contraceptive option in men. It is, however, used in a contraceptive pill for women, combined with oestrogen, because it is good at clearing up acne.

METHODS OF INHIBITING SPERM FUNCTION AFTER THEIR RELEASE

The irony of these methods is that they would have to be used by women. As mentioned earlier, sperm are still not fully functional until they are actually inside the woman's vagina, so it is possible to attack them there.

One possibility is a drug called propranolol, which is used in the treatment of high blood pressure. If the tablet is placed inside the vagina instead of swallowed, it appears to slow down the movement of sperm. Sperm cannot survive very long in the vagina itself because the environment is acidic (though they are very comfortable inside the womb and can live there for up to a week). If their stay in the vagina can be sufficiently prolonged, they will die.

A drug called sulphasalazine is used to treat a bowel condition called ulcerative colitis. One of its side effects is to reduce sperm motility and thus men taking it can become infertile. However, the effect is not seen in all the men who take it, and it is not easily reversible. This makes it unsuitable as a contraceptive, but scientists are looking at derivatives which might be more acceptable.

Another approach is to try and develop anti-sperm antibodies, which would destroy any sperm they meet. Such antibodies have been found in some infertile men, and also in some men after they have had a vasectomy (which reduces the success rates of vasectomy reversal). In these men, the antibodies literally destroy their own sperm. I have discussed the problems of trying to produce vaccines used by men, so once again it is likely that this would have the best chance of being effective if the antibodies were actually present in the woman, ready to attack sperm the minute they arrived.

OTHER IDEAS

It is well known that the testes are deliberately placed outside the main body in order for their temperature to be slightly lower than normal body temperature. Studies have shown that the production of sperm is reduced in hot weather, and a bright spark came up with the idea of 'scrotum warmers' to try and reduce fertility. You can imagine that this is neither very reliable, nor particularly comfortable or attractive.

The technique of vasectomy is not a hormonal method of contraception, and therefore is outside the scope of this book.

However, it is worth mentioning that research is going on to try and make vasectomy reversible, by putting plastic plugs into the tubes which it should later be possible to remove, hopefully with return of fertility.

IN CONCLUSION

As you can see, the prospect of a male hormonal method of contraception, let alone a 'male pill', is a very long way off. And even if it happened, it might have to be taken by women! However, the concept of greater male involvement in contraception generally is a good one which should be encouraged. If the need is not perceived to be there, funds will not be made available for research and a vicious circle ensues. But don't get excited yet.

10

THE PROS AND CONS OF HORMONAL CONTRACEPTION

Whenever hormonal contraception is mentioned, certain phrases almost immediately spring to mind: 'it's unnatural', 'tampering with nature', 'it's dangerous', and so on. It is rare to hear a woman make a positive remark. Most women, even if they use hormonal contraception, seem to be uneasy about it.

So how unnatural is hormonal contraception? As we have seen in this book, the majority of the methods rely to a greater or lesser extent on the prevention of ovulation, and it is this which women often think is so 'unnatural'. But, in fact, if you look into it, it is not natural at all for women to be constantly ovulating. In a society where family planning is not available, most sexually active women are always either pregnant or breastfeeding. In both of those conditions, periods disappear and therefore the woman is not ovulating. In fact, it is less than 100 years since the family of ten children (and we are not even counting the miscarriages) was commonplace in the UK. Those women married before they were 20, and may well have been pregnant almost every year until they were 35 or 40. During that time, because they were also breastfeeding, the chances are they had less than 10 or 20 periods – in 15 years.

Indeed, if you look at cancers of the breast, ovary and endometrium, they are all much less common in developing countries where large numbers of children and breastfeeding are still the norm. As we have seen, particularly in Chapter 2, these cancers seem to be related to the number of times a woman ovulates in her life, and methods of contraception which prevent ovulation, like the Combined Pill, offer considerable protection, at least against cancers of the ovary and endometrium.

So this worry about stopping ovulation is really unfounded: it could be argued that it is in fact far less 'natural' to prevent pregnancy while still ovulating.

Not that hormonal contraception is without risks or side effects. But neither is pregnancy, and one of the most important features of all hormonal methods is that they are very effective. If you compare the failure rates of hormonal and non-hormonal methods of contraception, only the intrauterine contraceptive device (IUD) is comparable (and how 'natural' is it to have a metal device inserted into your womb?) Barrier methods have failure rates in practice of between 10 and 15 per 100 women years. This means that out of 100 women using a diaphragm or sheath for a year, 10 to 15 are likely to become pregnant accidentally. If those same women used the pill, only one or at most two would become pregnant.

Methods which do not prevent ovulation improve with age, because older women ovulate less frequently anyway. For example women over 35 in general have more success using barrier methods. Young women, who are highly fertile, often do not realise that their failure rates in practice are likely to be higher than is often quoted in leaflets, since those are overall figures, which include older women.

If a method prevents ovulation, it does not matter if you are 16 or 60; if you don't ovulate, you will not become pregnant.

And there are other benefits to counter the possible risks. For example, period-related problems are often improved, which eases many women's lives. There are many other practical and health benefits to be gained from hormonal contraception, which I have discussed individually in relation to each method.

The pill has often been blamed for problems in society, ranging from the increase in sexually transmitted disease, to the removal of a woman's choice about whether or not to have sex. It is certainly true that without the pill the so-called 'sexual revolution' of the 1960s and 1970s might have been more difficult, but the trend had already become established before the pill became widely available. At first, women were simply taking more risks, and having what were then illegal abortions.

It is unfair to blame a method for the behaviour of some of the people who use it. The pill did not cause the increase in sexually transmitted disease, people did, by having larger numbers of partners. The sheath was first developed to prevent sexually transmitted disease, and there was nothing to stop couples using the pill as an effective contraceptive, while at the same time using the sheath to prevent the spread of infection. It has taken the fear of AIDS for this to be suggested as a reasonable thing to do.

Similarly, there have been allegations of the misuse of injectable progestogens in some developing countries and among some ethnic minorities. These led to an outcry that the method be banned. There is, in fact, little evidence to support this, but even if we assume that it may sometimes occur, it is surely the fault of the doctors or politicians involved, and not the method itself, which just happens to be a very effective and easy way to prevent pregnancy. Should all women be prevented from using safe and effective methods of contraception because of the possibility of misuse by or for a few?

Much more could be said about the political and social implications of all methods of contraception, but this book is primarily intended to present you with facts. Inevitably, anyone who works in the field of family planning, cervical screening, or sexually transmitted disease – and I have worked in all three – is bound to have their own views, which will to some extent colour the way the facts are presented. I expect I am just as guilty of this as all other authors, but I hope that this book has at least given you useful information, and some food for thought.

FURTHER READING

Below the Belt: A Woman's Guide to Genito-Urinary Infections, Denise Winn
Macdonald Optima, 1988

The Book of Love, Dr David Delvin
New English Library, 1975

The Breast Book, John Cochrane and Anne Szarewski
Macdonald Optima, 1989

The Cervical Smear Test: What Every Woman Should Know, Albert Singer and Anne Szarewski
Macdonald Optima, 1988

The Pill, John Guillebaud
Oxford University Press, 1984
A comprehensive guide to the Combined Pill and the Progestogen-Only Pill, written in terms anyone can understand. Written before much was known about the new Combined Pills, but a new edition is expected soon.

Contraception: Your Questions Answered, John Guillebaud
Pitman, 1985
A somewhat more technical look at all aspects of contraception.

Contraception: Science and Practice, Marcus Filshie and John Guillebaud
Butterworths, 1989
For the very interested, and those who have some scientific background. Written for doctors in the family planning field.

Private Parts: A Health Book for Men, Dr Yosh Taguchi
Macdonald Optima, 1988

Sexually Transmitted Diseases: The Facts, David Barlow
Oxford University Press, 1979

USEFUL ADDRESSES

UK

Association of Sexual and Marital Therapists
P.O. Box 62
Sheffield S10 3TS

British Association for Counselling
37a Sheep Street
Rugby, Warwickshire CV21 3BX
0788 78328
Useful source of nationwide information about clinics which provide counselling.

Brook Advisory Centres (Head Office)
233 Tottenham Court Road
London W1
071 323 1522/071 580 2991
Specialise in young people's problems (under 24). Provide family planning, screening services and counselling.

The Family Planning Association
27-35 Mortimer Street
London W1N 7RJ
071 636 7866
Gives advice on all aspects of family planning, sexual problems, etc. A good source of information about other clinics and services available throughout the United Kingdom. They have a bookshop and also free leaflets on many topics.

The Health Education Authority
Hamilton House
Mabledon Place
London WC1H 9TX
071 631 0930

Provides information and leaflets on all aspects of family planning.

Margaret Pyke Centre for Study and Training in Family Planning
15 Bateman's Buildings
Soho Square, London W1V 5TW
071 734 9351
The largest centre in Europe, dealing with all aspects of family planning, counselling and screening.

Relate (formerly National Marriage Guidance Council)
Head Office
Herbert Gray College
Little Church Street
Rugby, Warwickshire CV21 3AP
0788 73241
Nationwide network of clinics providing psychosexual and marriage guidance counselling. Local branches can be found in telephone directories.

Scottish Health Education Group
Woodburn House
Canaan Lane
Edinburgh EH10 4SG
031 447 8044
Similar to the above.

Scottish Marriage Guidance Council
26 Frederick Street
Edinburgh EH2 2JR
031 225 5006
Similar to Relate.

Terrence Higgins Trust
BM AIDS
London WC1N 3XX
071 833 2971/071 278 8745
Helpline 071 833 2971
Information, support groups and counselling about AIDS.

The Women's National Cancer Control Campaign
1 South Audley Street
London W1Y 5D
071 499 7532/4

Private family planning clinics

Hanway Clinic
1 Hanway Place
London W1P 9DF
071 636 0366

Marie Stopes House
The Well Women Centre
108 Whitfield Street
London W1
071 388 0662/2585

Marie Stopes Centre
10 Queen Square
Leeds LS2 8AJ
0532 440685

Marie Stopes Centre
1 Police Street
Manchester M4 7LQ
061 832 4250

EIRE

Irish Family Planning Clinic
Cathal Brugha Street
Dublin 1
Dublin 727276/727363
Provides a similar service to the FPA within the confines of Irish law.

UNITED STATES

Planned Parenthood Federation of America (head office)
2010 Massachusetts Avenue
NW Suite 500
Washington DC 20036
202 785 3351

Western region:
333 Broadway
3rd Floor
San Francisco
California 94133
415 956 8856

Southern region:
3030 Peachtree Road
NW Room 303
Atlanta
Georgia 30305

Northern region:
2625 Butterfield Road
Oak Brook
Illinois 60521
312 986 9270

AUSTRALIA

Australian Federation of FPAs
Suite 603, 6th floor
Roden Cutler House
24 Campbell Street
Sydney
NSW 2000

NEW ZEALAND

New Zealand FPA Inc.
PO Box 68200
214 Karangahape
Newton
Auckland

SOUTH AFRICA

FPA of South Africa
412 York House
46 Kerk Street
Johannesburg 2001

Pharmaceutical companies manufacturing hormonal contraceptives

These companies usually have information departments, which you may find helpful if you have a query relating to one or more of their products.

Gold Cross/Searle Pharmaceuticals
(Combined Pills: Conova 30; POPs: Femulen)
PO Box 53
Lane End Road
High Wycombe
Bucks HP12 4HL
0494 21124

Organon Laboratories Ltd
(Combined Pills: Marvelon, Mercilon, Minylin; combined oestrogen-progestogen vaginal ring; Desogestrel IUD)
Cambridge Science Park
Milton Road
Cambridge CB4 4FL
0223 423650

Ortho-Cilag Ltd
(Combined Pills: Neocon, Ovysmen, Ortho-Novin 1/50, Binovum, Trinovum, Trinovum ED; POPs: Micronor)
P.O. Box 79
Saunderton
High Wycombe
Bucks HP14 4HJ
024924 3541

Parke-Davis Medical
(Combined Pills: Loestrin 20, Loestrin 30)
Lambert Court
Chestnut Ave
Eastleigh
Hants SO5 3ZQ
0703 620500

Roussel Laboratories Ltd
(Progestogen-only vaginal ring)
Broadwater Park
North Orbital Road
Uxbridge, Middlesex UB9 5HP
0895 834343

Schering Health Care Ltd
(Combined Pills: Eugynon 30, Femodene, Microgynon,
Logynon, Logynon ED; POPs: Neogest, Norgeston; Post coital
pill: PC4; Injectable progestogen: Noristerat)
The Brow
Burgess Hill
West Sussex RH15 9NE
0444 232323

Syntex Pharmaceuticals Ltd
(Combined Pills: Brevinor, Norimin, Norinyl-1, Synphase;
POPs: Noriday)
Syntex House
St Ives Road
Maidenhead
Berks SL6 1RD
0628 33191

Upjohn Ltd
(Injectable contraceptive: Depo Provera)
Fleming Way
Crawley
West Sussex RH10 2NJ
0293 31133

Wyeth Laboratories
(Combined Pills: Minulet, Ovran, Ovran 30, Ovranette,
Trinordiol; POPs: Microval)
Huntercombe Lane South
Taplow
Maidenhead
Berks SL6 0PH
06286 4377

Huhtamaki Oy Leiras
(Levonorgestrel IUD; Norplant; Norplant 2)
P.O. Box 325 SF–00101
Helsinki
Finland
358 0 708811

INDEX

abortion, 26, 64, 86, 102, 103, 134
acne, 20, 36, 53, 95, 130
allergies, 55, 57–8
anaemia, 18
antibiotics, 41, 42, 56, 69, 70–1, 86, 90, 92, 99
antibodies, anti-sperm, 131
anti-emetics, 101
antifungal drugs, 69
arterial disease, 22, 23–4, 94
asthma, 57–8
atherosclerosis, 22, 23

bacteria: antibiotics, 41, 69–71, 86; and oestrogen levels, 69–71, 86
barbiturates, 69
barrier methods, 8, 100, 102, 104, 107, 134
bleeding *see* breakthrough bleeding; periods
blister packs, 61
bloating, 48, 58, 72, 80, 84
blood clots, 11, 21, 22, 64, 80, 93, 103
blood fats, 12–13, 14, 15, 23–5, 93–4, 108
blood pressure, 50–1, 74, 80, 93
blood sugars, 25, 79, 108
body hair, 52
bones, osteoporosis, 13, 110
brain: control of hormones, 1, 3–4, 5, 124, 127–9; stroke, 22, 49
breaks from the pill, 73
breakthrough bleeding, 40–6
breastfeeding, 30, 64, 80, 85, 92, 105–7, 115, 133
breasts: benign disease, 19, 30, 37; cancer, 20–1, 30–4, 80, 93, 96–8, 133; discharges from nipples, 47–8; enlargement, 46–7; tenderness, 36, 46–7, 80
Brevinor, 32, 43, 45, 46

cancer: breast, 20–1, 30–4, 81, 93, 96–8, 133; cervical, 28–30, 98; injectable progestogens and, 94, 95–8; liver, 26; ovarian, 20, 30, 93, 98, 133; Progestogen-Only Pill and, 81; uterus (endometrial), 20, 30, 93, 98, 110–11, 121, 133
candida, 56
capacitation, 7
Capronor, 119–20
carbamazepine, 69
cardiovascular disease, 13, 14, 21–5, 72, 80
carpal tunnel syndrome, 48
cervix: cancer, 28–30, 98; erosion, 55–6; mucus, 7, 8–9, 12, 13, 75–6, 85; smear tests, 29, 74
childbirth, taking pill after, 64, 86
chloasma, 53, 80
chloral hydrate, 69
chlorpromazine, 69
clinics, 74, 104
Combined Pill: benefits, 17–21, 34; breaks from, 73; changing to Progestogen-Only Pill, 84–5; development of, 10; functions, 8–9; for older women, 107–10; risks, 21–34; side effects, 35–59; taking, 60–74
condoms (sheaths), 8, 29, 100, 102, 104, 134–5
contact lenses, 54
corpus luteum, 4–5

145

Cotrimoxazole, 42
cramps in the legs, 57
Cyclo Provera, 121
cyproterone acetate, 130
cysts, ovarian, 18, 83, 92

deep vein thrombosis, 22–3, 25–6, 57
Depo Provera *see* injectable progestogens
depression, 51, 58, 80, 95, 111
desogestrel, 15, 24, 115, 121
diabetes, 25, 79
diaphragms, 8, 100, 102, 104, 134
diarrhoea, 67–8, 90
dichloralphenazone, 69
diet, and breast tenderness, 47
diosegenin, 9
discharges: from nipples, 47–8; vaginal, 55–6
diuretics, 69
doctors, 73–4, 104–5
drugs, interactions with the pill, 67–71, 87, 92
duodenal ulcers, 19

ectopic pregnancy, 7–8, 18, 83–4, 92, 103, 120
eczema, 57
ED (Every Day) preparations, 63, 67
egg *see* ovum
embryo, implantation, 7, 8, 76, 102
endometrial (uterine) cancer, 20, 30, 93, 98, 110–11, 121, 133
endometriosis, 19, 37, 72, 95
enzymes, liver, 41–2, 68–70, 86, 87, 99
epilepsy, 42, 67, 69, 73, 87, 92
Epilim, 68, 87
ergotamine, 49
ethinyloestradiol, 115
ethosuximide, 69
Eugynon, 32
eyes, contact lenses, 54

face, chloasma, 53, 80
failure rates: barrier methods, 134; Combined Pill, 60; hormone-releasing intrauterine devices, 120; implants, 117; injectable progestogens, 89; morning after pill, 102–3, 107;

Progestogen-Only Pill, 76–9, 110; vaginal rings, 114
fallopian tubes, 6, 7–8
Family Planning Association (FPA), 60
family planning clinics, 74, 104
fats, in diet, 47
Femodene, 38, 43–5, 47, 53, 69
Femulen, 78
fertilisation, 7, 8
fertility, 27, 80
fibroids, 19, 37
Follicle Stimulating Hormone (FSH), 1, 3, 5, 8, 124, 126, 129
follicles, 1–3
Food and Drug Administration (USA), 95, 96–7, 108, 113
forgotten pills, 41, 65–7, 84–5, 104
future developments, 113–22

gallstones, 57
gestodene, 15, 24
Gonadotrophin Releasing Hormone (GnRH), 1, 124, 128
gossypol, 129–30
greasy hair, 20, 36, 53, 95
griseofulvin, 69, 86

hair: benefits of Combined Pill, 20; greasy, 20, 36, 53, 95; hirsutism, 20, 36, 52, 84
headaches, 48–50, 58, 73, 80, 111
heart disease, 13, 21–5, 80, 110, 111
high-density lipoproteins (HDL cholesterol), 12–13, 14, 15, 23, 24, 72, 79, 93–4
hirsutism, 20, 36, 52, 84
hormone-releasing intrauterine devices, 120–1
hormone replacement therapy, 13, 110–11, 120–1, 122
hormones: development of hormonal contraception, 9–11; functions, 12–16; male, 124; natural, 1–8; pros and cons of hormonal contraception, 133–5; *see also* oestrogen; progestogen *etc.*
hospital casualty departments, 105
Human Chorionic Gonadotrophin (HCG), 4, 6, 26–7
human papillomavirus (HPV), 28–9
hydatidiform mole, 26–7
hypothalamus, 1, 124, 127–8

146

immune system, 57–8
implants, 111, 116–20
infertility, 18, 27
information leaflets, 60, 85
inhibin, 5, 121–2, 129
injectable progestogens: advantages, 91–4; breastfeeding and, 92, 105–6; and cancer, 94, 95–8; disadvantages, 94–5; ethics, 96, 135; functions, 89–90; future developments, 121; male contraception, 128; for older women, 110; starting and continuing, 99; types, 90–1; who should consider using, 99
intrauterine contraceptive devices (IUDs), 8, 102–3, 104, 107, 134; hormone-releasing, 120–1

jaundice, 26

legs, cramps, 57
levonorgestrel, 32, 113–14, 116, 120, 121
libido: loss of, 51–2, 80, 95; male, 124, 127, 128
liver: disease, 26; enzymes, 41–2, 67–9, 86, 87, 99, 112
Loestrin, 43–5, 46, 47
Logynon, 32, 43, 45, 63
low-density lipoproteins (LDL cholesterol), 13, 14, 23, 24
Luteinising Hormone (LH), 1, 4, 8, 66, 124, 126, 128, 129
Luteinizing Hormone Releasing Hormone (LHRH), 124

McCormick, Katherine, 10
male contraception, 7, 121–2, 123–32
Marvelon, 20, 38, 39–40, 43, 45–6, 53, 68
mastitis, 19
medicines, interactions with the pill, 67–71, 87, 92
medroxyprogesterone, 128
menopause, 13, 79, 93, 108, 110
menstrual cycle, 5, 12, 13
menstruation *see* periods
Mercilon, 38–40, 43, 45–6, 47, 53, 68, 110, 115
Microgynon, 32, 43, 45, 46, 47, 55
Micronor, 78

Microval, 78, 114
migraine, 48–50, 80
milky discharges, nipples, 47–8
mini-pill *see* Progestogen-Only Pill
Minulet, 38, 43–5, 47, 53, 68
Minylin, 63
miscarriage, 64, 85, 95
'mittelschmerz', 5–6
monilia, 56
monitoring health, 74
monophasic pills, 47, 49, 58
morning after pill, 67, 85, 100–5, 106
mucus, cervical, 7, 8–9, 12, 13, 75–6, 85

nasal sprays, 122, 128
natural hormones, 1–8
nausea, 54–5, 100
Neocon, 43–4, 46
Neogest, 78
neomycin, 69
nipples, milky discharge, 47–8
norethisterone, 32
norgestimate, 15, 24
Norgeston, 78
Noriday, 78
Norimin, 45
Noristerat, 91, 94, 99
Norplant, 116–19

oestradiol, 111
oestradiol cypionate, 121
oestrogen: and cardiovascular disease, 21–3; development of oral contraception, 10–11; dosages, 10, 11, 37–40; functions, 3–5, 12–13; hormone replacement therapy, 110–11, 121; for older women, 107–8, 111; patches, 122; side effects, 35–59; used with injectable progestogens, 94–5; vaginal rings, 115; *see also* Combined Pill
older women, 101–11
orgasm, 7
osteoporosis, 13, 110
ovaries: cancer, 20, 30, 93, 98, 133; cysts, 18, 83, 92; follicles, 1; forgotten pills, 65–7, 104; ovulation, 4, 5–6
Ovran, 32
Ovranette, 32, 43, 45, 46, 47, 55

147

ovulation, 4, 7; and cancer risks, 30, 93; forgotten pills, 65; injectable progestogens and, 89; morning after pill, 102; pain on, 5–6; Progestogen-Only Pill and, 75, 76, 81; as an unnatural event, 133–4
ovum: development of, 1–3; fertilisation, 7, 8; *see also* ovulation
Ovysmen, 32, 43, 45, 46

packaging, 61
patches, 122
pelvic inflammatory disease (PID), 8, 18, 92, 120
penicillin, 41, 69–71, 86
periods and withdrawal bleeding: after morning after pill, 102, and cancer risks, 20, 30, functions of withdrawal bleeds, 63, 72–3, with hormone-releasing intrauterine devices, 120; with implants, 118; and injectable progestogens, 92–3, 94–5; menstrual cycle, 5; missed withdrawal bleeds, 46; older women, 107–8; period pain, 18; post-pill amenorrhoea, 27; postponing, 71–2; Progestogen-Only Pill and, 81–2; with vaginal rings, 114, 115
pharmaceutical companies, 60, 142–3
phenytoin, 69
photosensitivity, 53
pituitary gland, 1, 3–4, 47–8, 124, 128–9
polycystic ovary syndrome, 18
pregnancy: after injectable progestogens, 92, 94; after morning after pill, 103; chloasma, 53; contraceptive failure rates, 60, 76–9, 89, 102–3, 107, 110, 114, 117, 120, 134; ectopic, 7–8, 18, 83–4, 92, 103, 120; hydatidiform mole, 26–7; and missed withdrawal bleeds, 46; in older women, 108; pregnancy tests, 6, 82; risks, 17–18; taking pill after, 64, 85; while taking the pill, 28; and withdrawal bleeds, 63
premenstrual syndrome (PMS), 18, 51, 54, 58–9, 93

primidone, 69
Progestasert, 120
progesterone: Combined Pill, 8; development of oral contraception, 9–11; functions, 4–5, 13–14; hormone-releasing intrauterine devices, 120; vaginal rings, 115
progestogen: and cardiovascular disease, 21–3; dosages, 11, 38; functions, 14–16; hormone replacement therapy, 110–11, 121; implants, 116–20; injectable, 89–99; for older women, 108; side-effects, 35–59; vaginal rings, 113–15; *see also* Combined Pill
Progestogen-Only Pill (POP): advantages, 79–80; breastfeeding and, 80, 105–6; changing to Combined Pill, 65; disadvantages, 80–4; effectiveness, 76–8; functions, 75–6; for older women, 110, 111; taking, 84–5; types, 78
prolactin, 5, 13, 47
propranolol, 131
pulmonary embolism, 11, 23

raised blood pressure, 50–1
rape, 100, 104
rheumatoid arthritis, 19, 58
'rhythm' method, 5
Rifampicin, 68, 69, 87
rings, vaginal, 113–15
rubella vaccine, 97

salpingitis, 8, 18, 92, 120
Sanger, Margaret, 10
'scrotum warmers', 131
sedatives, 69
Septrin, 42
sex: and cervical cancer, 28–9; dryness during, 52; loss of female libido, 51–2, 80, 95; male libido, 124, 127, 128; morning after pill, 100–5
Sex Hormone Binding Globulin (SHBG), 12, 14, 15, 32
sexually transmitted diseases, 134
sheaths (condoms), 8, 29, 100, 102, 104, 134–5
sickle cell disease, 92
side effects: Combined Pill, 10–11,

35–59; hormone replacement therapy, 111, 121; injectable progestogens, 94–5; morning after pill, 100–1; Progestogen-Only Pill, 80, 84
skin: acne, 20, 36, 53, 95, 130; benefits of Combined Pill, 20; chloasma, 53, 80; photosensitivity, 53
smoking, 21, 23–4, 29, 79, 107, 108, 110, 111
sodium valproate, 68, 69, 87
sperm: hormone control, 124; fertilisation of ovum, 7; life-span, 6; male contraception, 122, 127–31; production, 126–7; Progestogen-Only Pill and, 76
spermicides, 8, 57, 110
spironolactone, 69
sprays, nasal, 122, 128
steroids, 128
stomach upsets, 41, 67–8, 99, 112
stroke, 21, 22, 49
sugars, blood, 25, 79, 108
sulphasalazine, 131
sunbathing, 53
surgery, 25–6
systemic lupus erythematosus (SLE), 58

testes: male contraception, 129–30; temperature, 131
testosterone, 14, 126, 128
tests, pregnancy, 6, 82
tetracyclines, 41, 69–71, 86
thrombosis, 11, 22–3, 25–6, 64, 79, 93, 103
thrush, 56
Thunder God vine, 130
tranquillisers, 69
tricycling, 49, 73

Trinordiol, 32, 43, 45
Trinovum, 43, 45, 63
triphasic pills: postponing withdrawal bleeds, 71–2; side effects, 45, 47, 49, 51, 54, 58–9
tuberculosis, 42, 68, 87, 92

ulcers, duodenal, 19
'unisex' pills, 121–2, 129
uterus: breakthrough bleeding, 40; effects of progesterone, 4; endometrial cancer, 20, 30, 93, 98, 110–11, 121, 133; fibroids, 19; implantation of embryo, 7, 8, 76, 102; periods, 5; Progestogen-Only Pill and, 76, sperm in, 7

vaccines, male contraception, 129, 131
vagina: anti-sperm contraception, 131; discharges, 55–6; dryness, 52, 107; mucus, 7; thrush, 56
vaginal rings, 113–15
varicose veins, 26, 57
vasectomy, 131–2
vegetarians, 41
venous thrombosis, 11, 22–3, 25–6, 64, 80, 93, 103
vitamin B6, 47, 51
vitamin C, 42
vomiting, 67, 90, 100–1

water retention, 12, 14, 48, 54, 72
weight gain, 12, 14, 48, 79, 95
withdrawal bleeding *see* periods
withdrawal method, contraception, 7
womb *see* uterus

yams, 9
yeast infections, 56

More books from Optima

Cervical Smear Test by Albert Singer FRCOG and Dr Anne Szarewski
Recommended by the Family Planning Association
Every woman who has ever been sexually active is at risk from cervical cancer.

The majority who develop this disease have never had a smear test, a simple procedure designed to detect pre-cancerous cell changes, which can be literally life-saving.

This fully comprehensive and illustrated book, written by two experts in their field, is designed to provide information about cervical smear testing pertinent to every woman, her partner and her doctor. Using clear language it describes a cervical smear test, and what a 'positive' test means, colposcopy and its use; how abnormalities are treated; and cervical cancer and its causes and viruses. Psychological and emotional aspects are also covered.
ISBN 0 356 15065 8
Price (in UK only) £5.99

The Breast Book by John Cochrane MS FRCS and Dr Anne Szarewski
Recommended by the Family Planning Association
Every year thousands of anxious women consult their doctors about their breasts. Their anxieties range from suspected and actual lumps, premenstrual heaviness and tenderness, to dissatisfaction with their breasts' appearance.

Although the majority of breast problems are unrelated to cancer, and 80 per cent of all lumps are benign, for most women the underlying fear is that they may have breast cancer.

The Breast Book, written by two specialists, aims to dispel anxiety by providing accurate and reassuring information. Illustrated throughout, the book covers
- The structure and function of the breasts
- The importance of self-examination
- Breast lumps and breast cancer
- Breast problems in pregnancy and breastfeeding
- Cosmetic and reconstructive surgery
- Breast problems and the Pill
- Psychological and emotional aspects

ISBN 0 356 15416 5
Price (in UK only) £5.99

Understanding Endometriosis by Caroline Hawkridge
Endometriosis is an increasingly common gynaecological disorder, affecting an estimated one to two per cent of all women of childbearing age. Left untreated it is a chronic cause of pain, menstrual disorders and infertility.

In this book, written in conjunction with the Endometriosis Society and a medical expert, Caroline Hawkridge provides the most up-to-date summary of the disease and all that is known about its cause, diagnosis and treatment. Sympathetic and comprehensive, the book covers:
- Problems of diagnosis
- Managing pain
- Hormonal, surgical and alternative treatments
- Endometriosis and infertility
- Endometriosis and pregnancy
- Understanding your feelings

ISBN 0 356 15447 5
Price (in UK only) £5.99

Avoiding Osteoporosis by Dr Allan Dixon and Dr Anthony Woolf
Osteoporosis, or brittle bone disease, is the cause of pain and disability in one in four post-menopausal women in Britain. Yet this debilitating disease is preventable and treatable.

Dr Allan Dixon, Chairman of the National Osteoporosis Society, and Dr Anthony Woolf provide comprehensive and up-to-date information which is vital to all women and professionals concerned with the prevention of this disease.

The book covers:
- Causes and symptoms of osteoporosis
- Who is at risk
- Preventative measures during childhood, mid-life and old age
- Hormone Replacement Therapy and other treatments
- Practical guidance for safe and comfortable living

ISBN 0 356 15445 9
Price (in UK only) £5.99

All Optima books are available at your bookshop or newsagent, or can be ordered from the following address:

Optima, Cash Sales Department,
PO Box 11, Falmouth, Cornwall TR10 9EN

Please send cheque or postal order (no currency), and allow 60p for postage and packing for the first book, plus 25p for the second book and 15p for each additional book ordered up to a maximum charge of £1.90 in the UK.

Customers in Eire and BFPO please allow 60p for the first book, 25p for the second book plus 15p per copy for the next 7 books, thereafter 9p per book.

Overseas customers please allow £1.25 for postage and packing for the first book and 28p per copy for each additional book.